Cardiac Defibrillation
http://dx.doi.org/10.5772/45990
Edited by Damir Erkapic, Tamas Bauernfeind

ontributors
evin Michael, Damir Erkapic, Tamas Bauernfeind, Jorge Toquero, Dan Blendea, Craig McPherson, Razvan Dadu, arzia Giaccardi, Elisabete Martins, Joern Schmitt, Martin Seifert, Jerome Taieb, Munir Zaqqa

blished by InTech
za Trdine 9, 51000 Rijeka, Croatia

ocess Manager Iva Simcic
or InTech DTP team
esign team

pies can be obtained from orders@intechopen.com

n, Edited by Damir Erkapic, Tamas Bauernfeind

31-0

CAR
DEFIBRILLA

Edited by **Damir Erk**

Pu
Jan

Notice

Statements
of the edito
chapters. Th
use of any m

Publishing Pr
Technical Edit
Cover InTech D

Additional hard c

Cardiac Defibrillati
p. cm.
ISBN 978-953-51-09

Meet the editors

Dr. Erkapic finished medicine study at J.W. Goethe University of Medicine in Frankfurt/Main, approbation in 2006, at J. Gutenberg University of Medicine in Mainz, specialty in internal medicine, cardiology and electrophysiology at Kerckhoff Heart and Thorax Center in Bad Nauheim, J.W. Goethe University of Medicine in Frankfurt/Main and J. Liebig University of Medicine in Gießen (all in Germany). Currently Dr. Erkapic is Cardiologist/Electrophysiologist at the University Clinic of Gießen and Kerckhoff Heart and Thorax Center. Fellow of the German Heartrhythm Fellowship (2008-2010). He is member of the German Society of Cardiology (DGK), European Society of Cardiology (ESC) and European Heart Rhythm Association (EHRA). He is author and co-author of 2 books and several international publications in refereed journals and conferences.

Dr. Bauernfeind finished medicine study and approbation at Semmelweis University of Medicine 2003 in Budapest, specialty in internal medicine (2008) and cardiology (2011) following training at National Health Centre in Budapest, Thoraxcentre, Erasmus University in Rotterdam and Goethe University in Frankfurt/Main. Currently he is Consultant Cardiologist/Electrophysiologist at the Central Clinic of Suhl. Also, he is member of the Hungarian Society of Cardiology, German Society of Cardiology (DGK), and European Society of Cardiology (ESC). Dr. Bauernfeind is author and co-Author of several international publications in peer reviewed journals and conferences.

Contents

Preface

In highly developed countries, sudden cardiac death (SCD) caused by ventricular fibrillation or tachycardia (VF/VT) plays a prominent role in mortality since several decades. The invention of cardiac defibrillation proved to be a decisive step in the therapy and prophylaxis of SCD. As internal cardioverter defibrillator (ICD) therapy became widely available, a continuous development followed in the number and type of leads, programming capabilities and differential algorithms of these devices. Indications for ICD therapy also underwent consecutive changes and actualizations. However, several important issues concerning contraindications, possible complications, perioperative management including anticoagulation and antibiotic therapy, and the programming and follow-up of ICD devices are much less discussed in the available guidelines. In this book we tried to round up practical advices and protocols from colleagues working in the USA, Canada, Jordan, Portugal, Spain, France, Italy and Germany. We hope that you will find this book helpful for cardiologists and electrophysiologists to keep their knowledge "up-to-date".

Editor: Dr. Damir Erkapic, M.D.
University of Giessen and Marburg,
Kerckhoff Heart and Thorax Center,
Bad Nauheim, Germany

Co-editor: Dr. Tamas Bauernfeind, M.D.
SRH Zentralklinikum Suhl gGmbH
Internal Medicine I
Suhl, Germany

Section 1

External Cardiac Defibrillation

Chapter 1

Principles of External Defibrillators

Hugo Delgado, Jorge Toquero, Cristina Mitroi,
Victor Castro and Ignacio Fernández Lozano

Additional information is available at the end of the chapter

http://dx.doi.org/10.5772/52512

1. Introduction

Electrical defibrillation is the only effective therapy for cardiac arrest caused by ventricular fibrillation (VF) [1, 2] or pulseless ventricular tachycardia (VT). Scientific evidence to support early defibrillation is overwhelming [3-5], being delay from collapse to delivery of the first shock the single most important determinant of survival [6, 7]. If defibrillation is delivered promptly, survival rates as high as 75% have been reported [8, 9]. The chance of a favourable outcome decline at a rate of about 10% for each minute cardiac defibrillation is delayed [3, 10].

The guidelines on cardiopulmonary resuscitation of the European Resuscitation Council and American Heart Association (AHA) strongly recommend attempting defibrillation with minimal delay in victims of VF/VT cardiac arrest. As this event occurs most often in the victim's private home or in public spaces away from healthcare facilities, the need for early defibrillation has led to the development of automatic, portable defibrillators (Automated External Defibrillator - AED).

The purpose of this chapter is to review the mechanisms of external defibrillation, the available types of AEDs including the wearable cardioverter-defibrillator, its uses and limitations.

2. Cardiac external defibrillation – Basic science

2.1. History

In Switzerland, 1899, Prevost and Batelli discovered that small electric shocks could induce ventricular fibrillation in dogs and that larger charges would reverse the condition. However it was not until 1956 when alternating current was first used for transthoracic defibrillation to treat ventricular fibrillation in humans [11]. Following this breakthrough, direct current defibrillators were introduced into clinical practice around 1962 [12] when it was demonstrated that electrical countershock or cardioversion across the closed chest could abolish other cardiac arrhythmias in addition to ventricular fibrillation [13]. Later on, Diack et al. [14] described the first clinical experience with an AED. Subsequently, further studies provided solid evidence on the potential role of these devices in the early defibrillation and survival.

2.2. Types of defibrillators

- Most defibrillators are energy-based, meaning that the device charges a capacitor to a selected voltage and then delivers a prespecified amount of energy in joules. The amount of energy which arrives at the myocardium is dependent on the selected voltage and the transthoracic impedance (which varies by patient).

Most current AEDs are energy-based but there are two other types of defibrillators less frequently used in clinical practice.

- **Impedance-based defibrillators** allow selection of the current applied based upon the transthoracic impedance (TTI). TTI is assessed initially with a test pulse and subsequently the capacitor charges to the appropriate voltage. In patients with high TTI there was a significant improvement in shock success rate using this approach when compared to the energy-adjusting defibrillators [15].
- **Current-based defibrillators** deliver a fixed dose of current which results in defibrillation thresholds that are independent of TTI [16]. The optimal current for ventricular defibrillation appears to be 30 to 40 amperes independently of both TTI and body weight thus achieving defibrillation with considerably less energy than the conventional energy-based method [17-19]. Current-based defibrillation was proved superior to energy-based defibrillation with monophasic waveforms in one clinical study [20] but this concept merits further exploration in the light of biphasic waveforms now available.

2.3. Waveforms and its importance

Energy-based defibrillators can deliver energy in a variety of waveforms, broadly characterized as monophasic, biphasic or triphasic.

- **Monophasic waveform.** Defibrillators with this type of waveform deliver current in one polarity and were the first to be introduced. They can be further categorized by the rate at which the current pulse decreases to zero.If the monophasic waveform falls to zero gradually, the term damped sinusoidal is used. If the waveform falls instantaneously, the term truncated exponential is used *(figure 1)*.The damped sinusoidal monophasic waveforms have been the mainstay of external defibrillation for over three decades
- **Biphasic waveform.** This type of waveform was developed later. The delivered current flows in a positive direction for a specified time and then reverses and flows in a negative

http://dx.doi.org/10.5772/52512

direction for the remaining duration of the electrical discharge *(figure 2A)*. With biphasic waveforms there is a lower defibrillation threshold (DFT) that allows reductions of the energy levels administrated and may cause less myocardial damage [21-24]. The use of biphasic waveforms permits a reduction in the size and weight of AEDs.

- **Triphasic waveform.** There are no human studies to support the use of multiphasic waveforms over biphasic. Investigation in animals suggests that the benefits of biphasic waveform could be harnessed through the use of a triphasicwaveform in which the second phase has the larger strength to lower the DFT and the third phase the lower strength, to minimize damage [25] *(figure 2B)*.

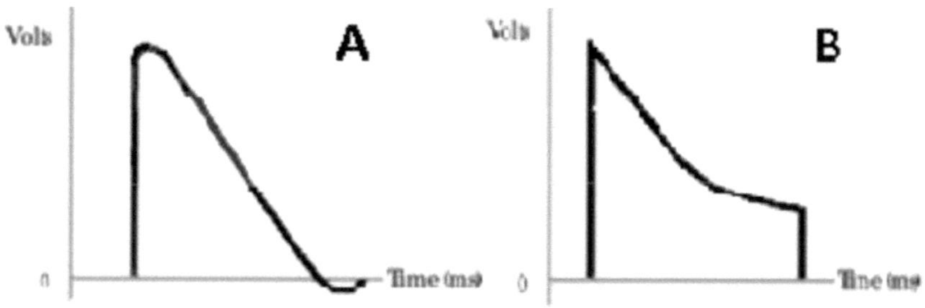

Figure 1. Monophasic waveforms. A. Damped sinusoidal wave (A) and truncated exponential (B).

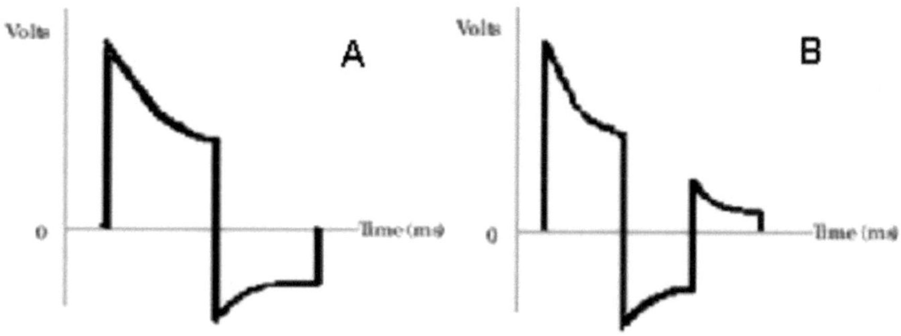

Figure 2. A. Biphasic waveform. B. Triphasic waveform.

2.4. Cardioversion and defibrillation

Cardioversion is one of the possible treatments for arrhythmias that imply a re-entrant circuit. By delivering a synchronized electric shock all excitable tissue of the circuit is simultaneously depolarised making the tissue refractory and the circuit no longer able to sustain reentry. As a result, cardioversion terminates arrhythmias resulting from a single reentrant circuit, such as atrial flutter, atrioventricular nodal reentrant tachycardia or monomorphic ventricular tachycardia. This term is also applied when using an electrical shock to terminate atrial fibrillation although this arrhythmia involves multiple, micro-reentrant circuits. The term cardioversion implies to syncronize the delivery of the shock with the QRS complex of the patient.

Defibrillation is used to describe the utilization of an electric shock to terminate ventricular fibrillation (VF). VF is known to be a very persistent arrhythmia, and total elimination of the fibrillatory activity is obtained only with a relatively high energy shock that uniformly depolarizes the entire myocardium.

Current European Society of Cardiology and AHA guidelines suggest the following initial energy selection for specific arrhythmias [26-28]:

- For atrial fibrillation, 120 to 200 joules for biphasic devices and 200 joules for monophasic devices.
- For atrial flutter, 50 to 100 joules for biphasic devices and 100 joules for monophasic devices.
- For ventricular tachycardia with a pulse, 100 joules for biphasic devices and 200 joules for monophasic devices.
- For ventricular fibrillation or pulseless ventricular tachycardia, at least 150 joules for biphasic devices and 360 joules for monophasic devices.

Cardioversion is most commonly used for the treatment of atrial fibrillation and the development of biphasic defibrillators proved to be very useful. At least 2 randomized trials illustrated the benefit of the biphasic waveform when compared to escalating monophasic shocks [29, 30]. First shock efficacy was greater with a biphasic waveform (68 versus 21 percent), delivered energy was 50 percent less, and the overall cardioversion rate was higher (94 versus 79 percent) [29]. There were fewer total shocks (1.7 versus 2.8), less energy delivered (217 versus 548 joules), and a lower frequency of dermal injury (17 versus 41 percent) [30].

Similar findings were reported for patients with atrial flutter, in whom cardioversion was successful more frequently and at lower energy levels when using biphasic waveforms [31].

3. Automatic external defibrillators

3.1. Definition and basic AED components

The term refers to a portable and lightweight computerized device that incorporates rhythm analysis and defibrillation systems and uses voice and/or visual prompts to guide lay rescuers and healthcare providers to safely defibrillate victims of cardiac arrest due to VF or pulseless VT.

There are two types of AED: the semi-automatic that indicates the need for defibrillation but requires that the operator deliver the shock by pushing a button and the fully automatic

http://dx.doi.org/10.5772/52512

AED which is capable of administering a shock without the need for outside interventions. See Table 1.

	Semi-automatic AEDs	Fully automatic AED
Definition	Indicates the need for defibrillation but requires an operator to deliver the shock by pushing a button	Capable of administering a shock without the need for outside interventions
Advantages	• Recommended by current resuscitation guidelines • Widely used • Allows healthcare professionals to override the device and deliver a shock manually, independently of prompts. • Safer, no risk of inappropriate shocks to the rescuer	• Easier to use and more appropriate for lay-rescuers • Better compliance with resuscitation protocols
Disadvantages	• More complex to use for the untrained responders • More difficult to synchronize with CPR maneuvers for lay rescuers	• Longer times until shock delivery • Risk of electrocution for the rescuer if inappropriately used • No possibility to override the device • Not recommended by current guidelines except for special situations

Table 1. Definition, main advantages and disadvantages for the different types of AED available.

Basically these devices consist of a battery, a capacitor, electrodes and an electrical circuit designed to analyze the rhythm and send an electric shock if is needed.

- **Batteries.** Essentially they are containers of chemical reactions and one of the most important parts of the AED system. Initially lead batteries and nickel-cadmium were used but lately non-rechargeable lithium batteries, smaller in size and with longer duration without maintenance (up to 5 years), are rapidly replacing them. Since extreme temperatures negatively affect the batteries, defibrillators must be stored in controlled environments. Also it is important to dispose of the batteries using designated containers as they contain corrosive and highly toxic substances.

- **Capacitor**. The electrical shock delivered to the patient is generated by high voltage circuits from energy stored in a capacitor which can hold up to 7 kV of electricity. The energy delivered by this system can be anywhere from 30 to 400 joules.

- **Electrodes** are the components through which the defibrillator collects information for rhythm analysis and delivers energy to the patient's heart. Many types of electrodes are available including hand-held paddles, internal paddles, and self-adhesive disposable electrodes. In general, disposable electrodes are preferred in emergency settings because they increase the speed of shock and improve defibrillation technique.

- **Electrical circuit**. AEDs are highly sophisticated, microprocessor-based devices that analyze multiple features of the surface ECG signal including frequency, amplitude, slope and wave morphology. It contains various filters for QRS signals, radio transmission and other interferences, as well as for loose electrodes and poor contact. Some devices are programmed to detect patient movement.
- **Controls.** The typical controls on an AED include a power button, a display screen on which trained rescuers can check de heart rhythm and a discharge button. Defibrillators that can be operated manually have also an energy select control and a charge button. Certain defibrillators have special controls for internal paddles or disposable electrodes.

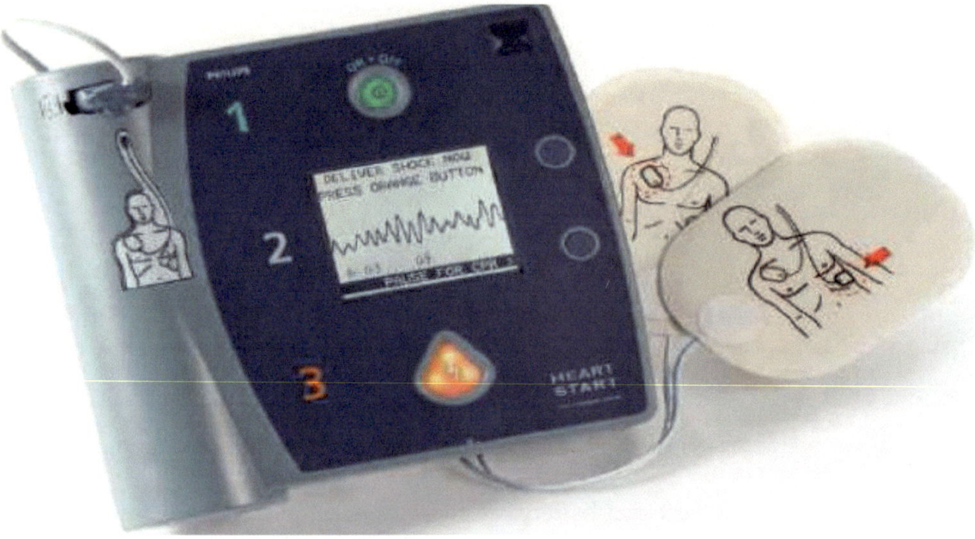

Figure 3. Appearance of a common AED with pads attached

3.2. Defibrillation success

Defibrillation is considered successful when it terminates VF for at least 5 seconds following the shock [32]. DFT is the lowest effective energy needed to restore the cardiac rhythm. Defibrillation basically depends on successful energy selection and TTI.

3.2.1. Energy levels

Modern AEDs are energy-based devices that can deliver the electrical shock in a monophasic or biphasic waveform. Although monophasic AEDs are not currently manufactured anymore they are still relatively easy to find in clinical practice. Energy levels vary by the type of device and the optimal energy level for defibrillation has not been determined yet.

Studies comparing biphasic shocks to a more traditional approach with 3 monophasic escalating shocks [33,34] have shown that defibrillation with relatively low energy (≤ 200 J biphasic) is safe and has equivalent or higher efficacy for termination of VF than monophasic waveform shocks of equivalent or higher energy [35-41]. However optimal energy for this first shock has not been determined so that for biphasic defibrillators, one should use the manufacturer's recommended energy dose (120 to 200 J). If the manufacturer's recommended dose is not known, defibrillation at maximal dose may be considered.

Commercially available biphasic AEDs provide either fixed or escalating energy levels. Human studies have not demonstrated evidence of harm from any biphasic waveform defibrillation energy up to 360 J [40, 41]. Based on available evidence, the second and subsequent shocks should be at an energy level equivalent or higher than the first one if possible.

In the absence of biphasic defibrillators, monophasic ones are acceptable. A recommendation for higher initial energy when using a monophasic waveform was weighed by expert consensus taking in consideration the potential negative effects of a high-energy first shock versus the negative effects of prolonged VF [42]. The consensus recommends that rescuers using monophasic AED should give an initial shock of 360 J. This single dose for monophasic shocks is designed to simplify instructions to rescuers but is not a mandate to recall monophasic AEDs for reprogramming. If the monophasic AED being used is programmed to deliver a different first or subsequent dose, that dose is acceptable.

3.2.2. *Transthoracic impedance*

It refers to the dissipation of energy in the lungs, thoracic cage and the other anatomic structures of the chest. In an animal study, only 4% of the energy supplied reached the heart [43]. The average adult human TTI is ≈70-80 Ω and is determined by multiple factors including energy level, electrode size, interelectrode distance, interface skin-electrode, electrode pressure, phase of ventilation, myocardial tissue and blood conductive properties [44].

When TTI is too high, a low-energy shock will not generate sufficient current to achieve defibrillation [44, 45]. To reduce TTI, the defibrillator operator should use conductive materials. This is accomplished with the use of gel pads or electrode paste [46] with paddles or through the use of self-adhesive pads.

3.2.3. *Others factors affecting defibrillation success*

There are several electrode characteristics that can affect defibrillation outcome. These include electrode position, pad size and hand-held versus patch electrodes. About electrode position, data demonstrates that 4 pad positions (antero-lateral, antero-posterior, anterior-left infrascapular and anterior-right-infrascapular) are equally effective [47].For ease of placement and education, antero-lateral is a reasonable default electrode placement. Electrode pad size is an important determinant of transthoracic current flow during external shock. Larger paddles create a lower resistance and allow more current to reach the heart [48, 49] and may cause less myocardial necrosis [50]. Thus, larger paddles are more desirable. Most manufacturers offer adult paddles, which are between 8 to 13 cm in diameter, and pediatric paddles, which are smaller [51].

Hand-held paddle electrodes may be more effective than self-adhesive patch electrodes because if applied with pressure they may improve electrode-to-skin contact and reduce TTI [52]. Nevertheless they are never used for AEDs because of the need for training.

3.3. Automated rhythm analysis

One of the most important features of an ideal AED is the accuracy of rhythm diagnosis. As demonstrated in both in vitro and clinical studies, accuracy in terms of sensitivity and specificity is high, surpassing 90% [53, 54]. The rare errors noted in trials occurred when the device failed to recognize certain varieties of VF or when operators failed to follow recommended instructions [54, 55]. In order to diagnose VF the device must identify an ECG waveform with amplitude of at least 0.8mV faster than a preprogrammed rate while for VT the criteria are: frequency of at least 120 beats/minute, QRS duration of more than 160 ms and absence of P wave. ECG analysis is done in consecutive segments of 2.7 seconds and the diagnosis must coincide in 2 out of 3 segments in order to give a decision.

Although AEDs are not designed to deliver synchronized shocks (such as cardioversion for VT with pulse), these devices will recommend a nonsynchronized shock for monomorphic or polymorphic VT if the rate and R-wave morphology exceed preset values. This is why AEDs should be placed in the analysis mode only when full cardiac arrest has been confirmed (patient unconscious) and all movement has ceased.

There is evidence that VF waveform analysis can predict defibrillation success rate. Several animal and model studies suggest that this analysis may help to identify the optimal timing or waveform for each patient [56, 57]. However this feature is not yet sufficiently accurate to be implemented in clinical practice.

3.4. Device maintenance and quality assurance

Appropriate maintenance of the AED is vital for proper operation. AED manufacturers provide specific recommendations for maintenance and readiness, which should be followed carefully. Failure to properly maintain the defibrillator or power supply is responsible for the majority of reported malfunctions. Newer AED models require almost no maintenance. These devices conduct a self-check of operation and indicate "readiness to use".

3.5. How to use an AED

3.5.1. Basic steps

AEDs are designed to be used by laypersons who ideally should have received AED training at some point in the past. Generally these devices are very intuitive and user-friendly so that even untrained bystanders can perfectly employ them to deliver an electric shock to a VF victim [58]. The basic steps common to all trademarks that need to be taken to deliver a shock are indicated in figure 4. In contrast, the more sophisticated manual and semi-automatic defibrillators used by health professionals can perform other functions but require a skilled operator able to interpret electrocardiograms.

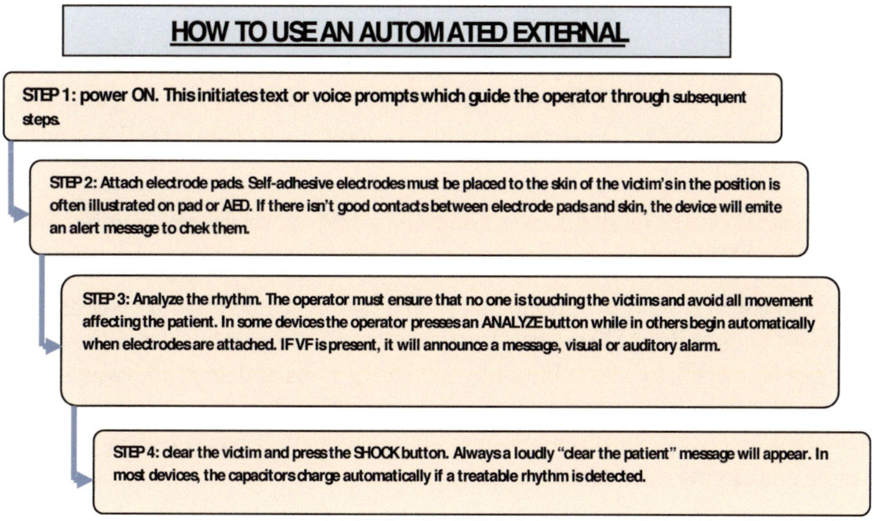

Figure 4. How to use an AED. Basic steps.

The location of a public access AED should be displayed to large groups of people, regardless of age or activity. In order to make them highly visible, public access AEDs are often brightly colored, and are mounted in protective cases near the entrance of a building. In September 2008, the International Liaison Committee on Resuscitation issued a 'universal AED sign' to be adopted throughout the world to indicate the presence of an AED (figure 5).

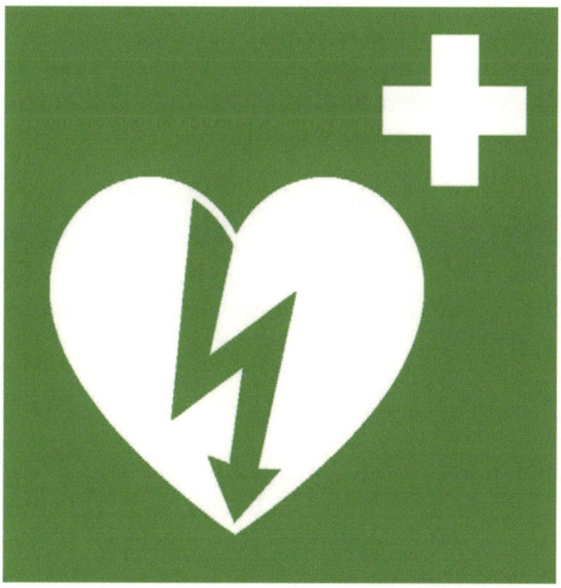

Figure 5. Universal AED sign

3.5.2. Integration of AED use with basic life support measure

When arriving at the scene of a suspected cardiac arrest, rescuers must rapidly integrate cardiopulmonary resuscitation (CPR) with the use of the available AED. In general 3 actions must occur simultaneously: (1) activation of the Emergency System, (2) CPR and (3) operation of the AED (figure 6).

Latest European Resuscitation Council Guidelines [59] emphasize a number of changes compared to the 2005 version:

- Chest compression should be initiated as soon as possible and should be continued while the adhesive pads of the AED are being attached and during defibrillator charging. If only one rescuer is present, he should initially attach the pads and start afterwards chest compressions. With a sole rescuer present, it is recommended to do only chest compressions with no ventilation. If 2 or more rescuers are present chest compression and ventilation should be done in the classical 30:2 sequence.
- Minimize interruptions in CPR. The importance of early, uninterrupted chest compression is emphasized in all guidelines. Interrupt CPR only when it is necessary to analyze the rhythm and deliver a shock. The delivery of defibrillation should be achievable with an interruption in chest compressions of no more than 5 seconds. After an electrical shock it is recommended to start CPR immediately for the next 2 minutes and only after that stop to reanalyze the cardiac rhythm
- In the previous version of guidelines, CPR was recommended for 2-3 minutes before analyzing a rhythm. Now this recommendation was withdrawn for lack of benefit.
- The previous recommendation for three-stacked shocks is also withdrawn for the out-of-hospital VF. This strategy should be employed only with witnessed VF in the hospital setting such as in the cath-lab or for patients with recent heart surgery. All cardiac arrests in out-of-hospital setting should be treated with an initial shock if found in VF followed by 2 minutes CPR and subsequent rhythm reanalysis.
- Electrode pastes and gels can spread between the two paddles, creating the potential for a spark and should not be used.

Modified prototype AEDs record information about frequency and depth of chest compressions during CPR. These devices are now commercially available and can prompt rescuers to improve CPR performance.

3.5.3. AED use in pediatric and adolescent population

Cardiac arrest is less common in children than adults. In pediatric population cardiac arrest causes are more diverse with only 5% to 15% of all cases being attributed to VF [60]. The lowest-energy dose for effective defibrillation and upper limit for safe defibrillation in infants and children are not known, but doses > 4 J/kg have effectively defibrillated children [61] and pediatric animal models [62]. Biphasic shocks appear to be at least as effective as monophasic shocks and less harmful, initial doses of 2 J/kg may be considered. Some AEDs are equipped with pediatric attenuator systems to reduce the delivered energy to a dose suitable for children [63]. It seems that most AEDs can accurately detect VF in children with a high degree of sensitivity and specificity, but more studies are needed.

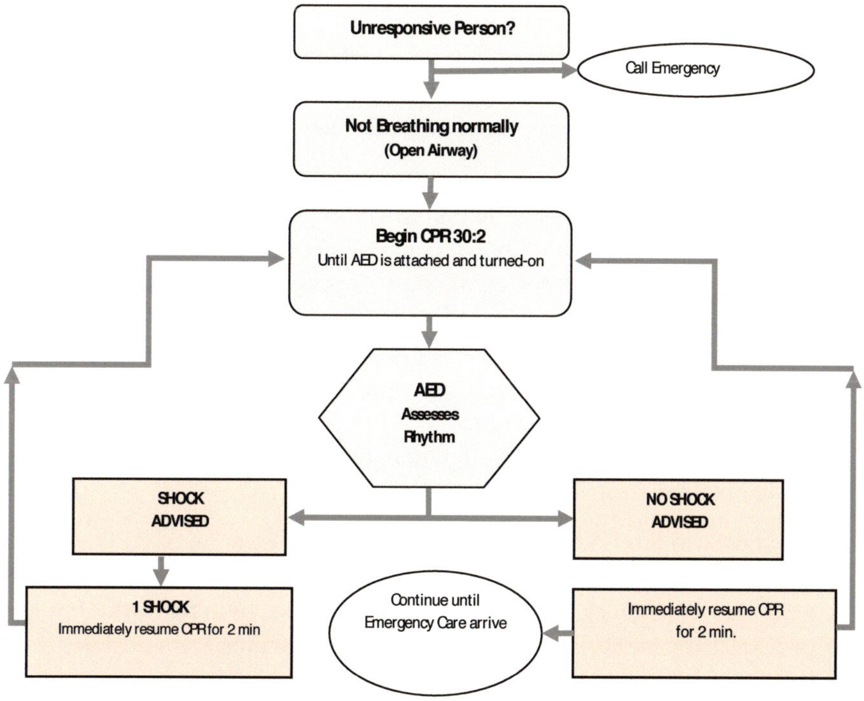

Figure 6. AED and CPR algorithm.

European and AHA guidelines recommend the using conventional, adults AEDs in children > 8 years old (approximately 25 kg body weight) with the same energy recommendation as in adult population. In children < 8 years it is reasonable to use a pediatric dose-attenuator system but if none is available the rescuer should use a standard AED. Infants should be treated with manual or dose-attenuating defibrillators although there are isolated cases of adult AED use in infants with good outcomes and without apparent myocardial damage [64].

3.6. AED for the masses

3.6.1. AED use training

The design of AEDs is centered on being easy to use even for the untrained lay rescuers. A variety of studies have demonstrated that it is feasible especially when the rescuers receive instructions via telephone from emergency dispatchers [65, 66]. However, in order to improve outcomes in out-of-hospital cardiac arrests, the 'ideal' rescuer should have minimal training on AED use and basic CPR. Multiple approaches for AED training and maintenance of learned skills have been employed (face-to-face, video or web-based training) with various degrees of success [67, 68].

3.6.2. Public access defibrillation

This concept includes all those strategies or programs to implement early defibrillation in the community. It has emerged from the recognition that AEDs and training lay people to use it are promising methods to achieve rapid defibrillation and survival in out-of-hospital cardiac arrest.

Resuscitation guidelines recommend early defibrillation (within 5 minutes of collapse) in order to increase survival from out-of-hospital cardiac arrest. The only way to achieve this goal is by generalizing of AEDs in the community. It is now accepted than an AED should be available for immediate use by trained laypersons wherever large numbers of people congregate [69, 70] such as airports, convention centers, sports stadiums and arenas, large industrial buildings, high-rise offices, large health fitness facilities. Furthermore AED should be provided also to the traditional emergency medical services (EMS), to non-medical emergency responders (police officers and firefighters), as well as placed in hospitals and in the private homes of high-risk individuals.

- **AED use by EMS.** In the USA initial large scale implementation of AED was with EMS and took place in the 1980s and 1990s. This strategy allowed EMS first responders, many of them who were emergency medical technicians without training in rhythm interpretation, to provide early defibrillation to cardiac arrest victims.Meta-analyses found that EMS AED programs resulted in a significant, overall 9 percent increase in survival [71, 72] although not all of the individual reports showed survival advantage [73].One plausible explanation for this discrepancy is that the resuscitation algorithms originally used for AED rhythm analysis required considerable interruptions in CPR [74], and that the increase in "hands-off" time reduced the chances of successful resuscitation [75]. More recent AED algorithms and guideline recommendations for minimally interrupted cardiac resuscitation have demonstrated improved outcomes for out-of-hospital cardiac arrest victims [76, 77].

- **AED use by police officers and firefighters** was implemented in various USA states. Policemen were provided with AED and trained how to use them. Several studies demonstrated that this approach was able to significantly increase survival to hospital discharge and without neurological deficits [78, 79]. However this advantage was evident only in those states where police officers were able to get to the victim before EMS emphasizing one more time the importance of early defibrillation.

- **AED use in private homes** is a strategy that seems useful sincethree-quarters of sudden cardiac arrests occur in the victim's home. This approach was investigated by a randomized trial that included 7001 patients with previous anterior wall myocardial infarction who were not candidates for an implantable cardioverter-defibrillator [80]. There was no survival benefit for AED and CPR group versus CPR only. The negative result may be ex-

http://dx.doi.org/10.5772/52512

plained by a lower than expected cardiac arrest rate with only 50% of the events being witnessed and by a low usage of AED (only in 32 victims out of 117). In deciding whether AEDs are appropriate for home use, cost and the increasing role of implantable cardioverter-defibrillators in high risk individuals must be taken into consideration.

- **AED use in hospitals** was studied because of data suggesting thatdelayed defibrillation is common during in-hospital arrest even though medical personnel are often trained in rhythm interpretation and manual defibrillation. A delay of more than 2 minutes between collapse and defibrillation was associated with a lower probability of survival [81]. While small studies with AED allocated to specific clinical and non-clinical areas of the hospital suggested improved survival [82, 83], large registry data showed discrepant results [84]. Patients with in-hospital cardiac arrest by VF/pulseless VT reanimated using an AED had the same survival rate as those who were not treated with these devices. The patients with cardiac arrest without a shockable rhythm (asystole or pulseless electrical activity) had significantly worse survival when an AED was used, probably because of delays/interruptions in CPR needed for AED rhythm analysis. The optimal strategy of AED distribution and its ultimate benefit may depend upon a particular hospital's staffing, geography, and patient profile.

- **Survival benefit and cost efficiency in public access defibrillation**

- Several clinical, randomized, prospective studies confirmed a robust survival benefit when victims of cardiac arrest in public places where reanimated by lay rescuers who did CPR and used an AED versus CPR only. The survival rate to discharge was 23.4%when an AED was used versus 14% with CPR only in PAD trial [85] and 38% versus 9% in the largest cohort of patients that included 13.000 individuals [86]. Cost efficiency analysis showed a cost of $35,000 to $57,000 per quality adjusted life-year [87, 88], which is comparable to other widely-accepted medical interventions such as bone marrow transplant ($52,000 per quality adjusted life-year) and heart transplant ($59,000 per quality adjusted life-year). So convincing was the evidence of AED benefit that USA authorities established rules to implement AED programs in schools and many other federal locations [89].

3.7. Wearable cardioverter-defibrillator

3.7.1. Definition and indications

The wearable cardioverter-defibrillator (WCD) (LifeVest®, ZOLL) is an external device capable of automatic detection and defibrillation of VT and VF. Its main indication is in situations where implantable cardioverter-defibrillator (ICD) may be initially deferred or may become unnecessary if the arrhythmic substrate is temporary or if the risk of ICD implantation is too high. While the WCD can be worn for years, typically the device is used for several months as temporary protection against cardiac arrest. The main indications were a WCD may be used are as follows:

- Recent myocardial infarction or coronary revascularization with severely reduced left ventricular ejection fraction

- Newly diagnosed nonischemic cardiomyopathy with severely reduced left ventricular ejection fraction
- Severe cardiomyopathy as a bridge to heart transplantation or in patients with ventricular assist devices
- Need for interruption of ICD therapy or the temporary inability to implant an ICD (e.g. infection)
- Syncope and a high risk of ventricular tachyarrhythmias
- Ambulatory event monitoring, often performed for several weeks in an effort to determine an arrhythmic etiology for syncope

3.7.2. How a WCD works

This device is composed of four non adhesive monitoring electrodes, three defibrillation electrodes incorporated into a chest strap assembly and positioned for apex-posterior defibrillation and a defibrillation unit carried on a waist belt. The monitoring electrodes must be placed circumferentially around the chest and held in place with an elastic belt. They provide 2 surface ECG leads. It is essential that the vest be properly fitted in order to have adequate skin contact and avoid noise and frequent alarms. See figure 7.

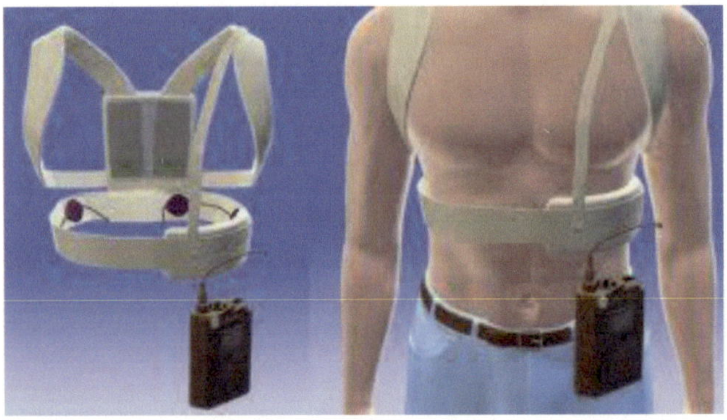

Figure 7. LifeVest®, ZOLL: main components and how it should be worn.

Arrhythmia detection by the WCD is programmed using rate criteria. When an arrhythmia is detected, the WCD emits audible and vibration alarms. The patients are trained to hold response buttons during these alarms in order to avoid a shock while awake. If an electric shock will be delivered a voice cautions the patient and bystanders to the impending shock. A patient's response serves as a test of consciousness; if no response occurs, the device charges, extrudes gel from the defibrillation electrodes, and delivers up to five biphasic shocks at preprogrammed energy levels with a maximum output of 150 joules.

http://dx.doi.org/10.5772/52512

The tachycardia detection rate is programmable for VF between 120 and 250 beats/minute and the VF shock delay can be programmed from 25 to 55 seconds. The VT detection rate is programmable between 120 bpm to the VF setting with a VT shock delay of 60 to 180 seconds. Additional shock delays (up to 30 seconds) may optionally be allowed during sleep. VT signals can allow synchronized shock delivery on the R wave, but if the R wave cannot be identified, unsynchronized shocks will be delivered. The shock energy is biphasic and can be programmed from 75 to 150 joules, with up to five shocks delivered per event.

The WCD has also the capability to store data regarding arrhythmias or asystole, patient's compliance with the device, noise and interference. All this information is stored and later transmitted via modem to the manufacturer network where it is available for clinician review. Of note is that WCD cannot deliver either antitachycardia pacing or pacing for bradycardia or asystole. (cannot + either/or vs. can + neither/nor)

3.7.3. Efficacy of WCD and other aspects

In the USA postmarket study of 3569 patients, there were 80 sustained VT/VF events that occurred and the success of the first shock in terminating VT/VF in the unconscious patients was 100% with a survival rate of 86%. Death after a successful first shock occurred because recurrent VT/VF, bystander preventing therapy in one case, electrocardiogram signal disruption from a fall, and to inhibition of detection due to the pacing stimulus artifact from a unipolar pacemaker (one case). This study also reported that long-term survival was similar in WCD patients compared to a cohort of ICD patients [90]. Nevertheless, WCD does not offer pacemaker functions and in this study 23 out of 3569 patients (0.6%) experienced asystole with an associated mortality of 74%

Although the WCD is a very efficient device, cardiac arrest still can develop in some circumstances: patient does not wear the device, WCD is improperly positioned, or bystander interference. These results highlight the importance of patient education and compliance while using the WCD.

Some of the shocks that a WCD delivers may be inappropriate due to electronic noise, malfunction of the device or supraventricular tachycardia. The rate of inappropriate shocks by a WCD is comparable to the ICD rate [90, 91]. However WCD inappropriate shocks can be potentially reduced due to the ability to abort shock by pressing response buttons if the patient is awake. Also, when ECG noise occurs, the device emits an alarm prompting the patient to try to eliminate the electronic noise by changing body position or tightening of the electrode belt.

In spite of being an extremely efficient device, WCD has some important limitations that need to be acknowledged. It does not provide pacemaker functions and it requires patient interaction and compliance. The device must be removed for bathing and during this time periods a caregiver should be present. In one German study [91], mean daily use of WCD was 21.3 hours/day. The primary complaints associated with the WCD were the weight of the device, problems sleeping, particularly when noise alarms occurred and skin rash or itching.

3.8. Legal issues concerning AED

In the past use of AEDs was limited partly because of the concern for subsidiary responsibility of those who are not health personnel. The fact that defibrillation is a medical act represents a legal obstacle in many countries. In 2000 the U.S. Congress approved the Act of survival in cardiac arrest, which extended the protection of the Good Samaritan to the users of an AED. Lay rescuers are protected from lawsuits if they act voluntarily to try to help a person who is having a medical emergency. The rescuer should act with good faith and make an effort help another person The rescuer's efforts must be reasonable and with common sense. This has been an important step in the diffusion and generalization of these devices.

3.9. Challenges and future development for AED

While these devices are very effective when treating ventricular arrhythmias, they still the need the presence of a bystander capable of applying and operating it. Also, it must be taken into account, that only a half of the cardiac arrests are witnessed so for a large number of patients this therapy cannot be available.

The main drawback that was observed when using an AED is that it requires interruptions in CPR in order to analyze the rhythm and to deliver the electric shock.Ongoing efforts are aimed at minimizing this time, and technical advances may eventually enable accurate rhythm interpretation even while CPR is ongoing [92, 93]. Recent resuscitation guidelines emphasize strongly the need to reduce 'hands-off' time in order to obtain a favorable result.

It was advocated that AED should be included in the category of compulsory safety equipment such as smoke alarms or fire extinguishers. However this approach has not demonstrated survival benefit and at the moment is cost prohibitive.

One of the future directions of research is AED analysis of shape and pattern of VF waveform recorded by ECG. It promises help in guiding the rescuers for the best course of treatment with CPR, defibrillation and medication. See section 3.3

4. Conclusions

Sudden cardiac arrest, frequently due to VF or pulseless VT, is traditionally associated with poor survival rates. Saving the lives of these patients depends on early cardiac defibrillation which, with manual defibrillators, is limited only to qualified rescuers who can interpret ECGs. AEDs solve this problem since they are able to analyze rhythm and inform the rescuers whether a shock is indicated. This approach allows lay rescuers to provide effective early defibrillation which has been shown to significantly improve survival and survival with intact neurologic function after out-of-hospital cardiac arrest. One limitation is that AED use requires interruptions in CPR which was proved to be deleterious especially in patients with non-shockable rhythms. Special efforts are being made in order to improve rhythm analysis and 'hands-off' time during CPR.

Author details

Hugo Delgado, Jorge Toquero*, Cristina Mitroi, Victor Castro and Ignacio Fernández Lozano

*Address all correspondence to: jorgetoquero@secardiologia.es

Hospital Puerta de Hierro Majadahonda, Madrid, Spain

References

[1] White RD. EMT-defibrillation:time for controlled implementation of effective treatment. AHA Emergency Cardiac Care Newsletter.1986;8:1-3.

[2] Swor RA, Jackson RE, Cynar M, sadler E, Basse E, Boji B, River-Rivera EJ, Maher A, Grubb W, Jacobson R, Dalbec DL. Bystander CPR ventricular fibrillation, and survival in witnessed, unmonitored out-of-hospital cardiac arrest. Ann Emerg. Med. 1995;25:780-784.

[3] Eisenberg MS, Horwood BT, Cummins RO, Reynolds-Haertle R, Hearne TR. Cardiac arrest and resuscitation: a tale of 29 cities. Ann Emerg Med.1990;19:179-186.

[4] Larsen MP, Eisenberg MS, Cummins RO, Hallstrom AP. Predicting survival from out-of-hospital cardiac arrest: a graphic model. ANnnEmerg Med.1993;22:1652-1658.

[5] Weaver WD, Copass MK, Bufi D, Ray R, Hallstrom AP, Cobb LA. Improved neurologic recovery and survival after early defibrillation. Circulation.1984;69:943-948.

[6] Eisenberg MS, Copass MK, hallstrom AP, blake B, Bergner L, Short FA, Cobb LA. Treatment of out-of-hospital cardiac arrest with rapid defibrillation by emergency medical technicians. N Engl J Med.1980;302:1379-1383.

[7] Cummins RO. From concept to standard-of-care? Review of the clinical experience with automated external defibrillations. Ann Emerg Med. 1989;18:1269-1275.

[8] Wik L, Hansen TB, Fylling F, Steen T, Vaaagenes P, Auestad BH, Steen PA. Delaying defibrillation to give basic cardiopulmonary resuscitation to patients with out-of-hospital ventricular fibrillation: a randomized trail. JAMA.2003;289:1389-1395.

[9] Cobb LA, Fahrenbruch CE, Walsh TR, Copass MK, Olsufka M, breskin M, Hallstrom AP. Influence of cardiopulmonary resuscitation prior to defibrillation in patients with out-of-hospital ventricular fibrillation. JAMA 1999;281:1182-1188.

[10] Holmberg M, Holmberg S, Herlitz J. Incidence, duration and survival of ventricular fibrillation in out-of-hospital cardiac arrest patients in Sweden. Resuscitation. 2000;44:7-17.

[11] Zoll PM, Linenthal AJ, Gibson W, et al. Termination of ventricular fibrillation in man by externally applied electric countershock. N Engl J Med 1956; 254:727.

[12] Lown B, Amarasingham R, Neuman J. New method for terminating cardiac arrhythmias. Use of synchronized capacitor discharge. JAMA 1962; 182:548.

[13] Zoll PM, Linentha AJ. Termination of refractory tachycardia by external countershock. Circulation 1962; 25:596.

[14] Diack AW, Welborn WS, Rullman RG, Walter CW, Wayne MA. An automatic cardiac resuscitator for emergency treatment of cardiac arrest. Med Instrum.1979;13:78-83.

[15] Kerber, RE, Martins, JB, Kienzle, MG, et al. Energy, current, and success in defibrillation and cardioversion: Clinical studies using an automated impedance-based method of energy adjustment. Circulation 1988; 77:1038.

[16] Kerber, RE, Jensen, SR, Gascho, JA, et al. Determinants of defibrillation: Prospective analysis of 183 patients. Am J Cardiol 1983; 52:739.

[17] Lerman, BB, DiMarco, JP, Haines DE. Current-based versus energy-based ventricular defibrillation: A prospective study. J Am CollCardiol 1988; 12:1259.

[18] Schönegg M, Schöchlin J, Bolz A. Patient-dependent current dosing for semi-automatic external defibrillators (AED). Biomed Tech (Berl). 2002;47Suppl 1 Pt 1:302-19. Lerman BB, Dimarco JP, Haines DE. Current-based versus energy based ventricular defibrillation: a prospective study. J Am collcardiol. 1988;12;1259-1264.

[19] Kerber RE, Kieso RA, Kienzle MG, Olshansky B, Waldo AL, Carlson MD, Wilber DJ, Aschoff AM, birger S, Charbonnier F. Current-based transthoracic defibrillation. Am J Cardiol.1996;78:1113-1118.

[20] Cummins RO, Hazinski MF, et Al. Low-energy biphasic waveform defibrillation:evidence-based review applied to emergency cardiovascular care guidelines: a statement for healthcare professionals from the AHA. Circulation 1998;97:1654-1667.

[21] Fain E, Sweeney m, Et Al. Improved internal defibrillation efficacy with a biphasic waveform. Am. Heart J. 1989; 117:358-364.

[22] Chapman PD, Vetter JW, Souza JJ, Comparative efficacy of monophasic and biphasic truncated exponential shocks for nonthoracotomy internal defibrillationin dogs. J Am CollCardiol. 1988;12:739-745.

[23] Cates AW, Souza JJ, Hillsley, Et Al. Probability of defibrillation success and incidence of postshock arrhythmias as a function of shock strength. J Am CollCardiol. 1993;21:21:305.

[24] Zhang Y, Ramabadran RS, Bodicker KA, et al. Triphasic waveforms are superior to biphasic waveforms for transthoracic defibrillation: experimental studies. J Am Coll-Cardiol 2003;42:568-574.

[25] Fuster V, Rydén LE, Cannom DS, et al. ACC/AHA/ESC 2006 Guidelines for the Management of Patients with Atrial Fibrillation: a report of the American College of Cardiology/American Heart Association Task Force on Practice Guidelines and the

European Society of Cardiology Committee for Practice Guidelines (Writing Committee to Revise the 2001 Guidelines for the Management of Patients With Atrial Fibrillation): developed in collaboration with the European Heart Rhythm Association and the Heart Rhythm Society. Circulation 2006; 114:e257.

[26] Zipes DP, Camm AJ, Borggrefe M, et al. ACC/AHA/ESC 2006 Guidelines for Management of Patients With Ventricular Arrhythmias and the Prevention of Sudden Cardiac Death: a report of the American College of Cardiology/American Heart Association Task Force and the European Society of Cardiology Committee for Practice Guidelines (writing committee to develop Guidelines for Management of Patients With Ventricular Arrhythmias and the Prevention of Sudden Cardiac Death): developed in collaboration with the European Heart Rhythm Association and the Heart Rhythm Society. Circulation 2006; 114:e385.

[27] Link MS, Atkins DL, Passman RS, et al. Part 6: electrical therapies: automated external defibrillators, defibrillation, cardioversion, and pacing: 2010 American Heart Association Guidelines for Cardiopulmonary Resuscitation and Emergency Cardiovascular Care. Circulation 2010; 122:S706.

[28] Mittal S, Ayati S, Stein KM, et al. Transthoracic cardioversion of atrial fibrillation: comparison of rectilinear biphasic versus damped sine wave monophasic shocks. Circulation 2000; 101:1282.

[29] Page RL, Kerber RE, Russell JK, et al. Biphasic versus monophasic shock waveform for conversion of atrial fibrillation: the results of an international randomized, double-blind multicenter trial. J Am CollCardiol 2002; 39:1956.

[30] Mortensen K, Risius T, Schwemer TF, et al. Biphasic versus monophasic shock for external cardioversion of atrial flutter: a prospective, randomized trial. Cardiology 2008; 111:57.

[31] White RD. External defibrillation: the need for uniformity in analyzing and reporting results (editorial). Ann Emerg. Med.1998;32:234-236.

[32] Kudenchuk PJ, Cobb LA, Copass MK, Olsufka M, Maynard C, Nichol G. transthoracic incremental monphasic versus biphasic defibrillation by emergency responders (TIMBER): a randominized comparison of monophasic with biphasic waveform ascending energy defibrillation for the resuscitation of out-of-hospital cardiac arrest due to ventricular fibrillation. Circulation. 2006;114:2010-2018.

[33] Leng CT, Paradis NA, calkins H, Berger RD, Lardo AC, Rent KC, Halperin HR. Resuscitation after prolonged ventricular fibrillation with use of monophasic and biphasic waveforms pulses for external defibrillation. Circulation.2000;101;2968-2974.

[34] Alem AP, Chapman FW, Lank P, Hart AA, koster RW, A prospective, randomized and blinded comparison of first shock success of monophasic and biphasic waveforms in out-of-hospital cardiac arrest. Resuscitation.2000;58:17-24.

[35] Morrison LJ, Dorian O. long J, Vermeulen M, Schwarts B, sawadsky B, Frank J, Cameron B, Burgess R, Shield J. Out-of-hospital cardiac arrest rectilinear biphasic to monophasic damped sine defibrillation waveforms with advanced life support intervention trial (ORBIT). Resuscitation.2005;66:149-157.

[36] Carpenter j, Rea TD, Murray JA, Kudenchuck PJ, Eisenberg MS. Defibrillation waveform and post-shock rhythm in out-hospital ventricular fibrillation cardiac arrest. Resuscitation.2003;59:189-196.

[37] Stohert JC, hatcher TS, Gupton CL, love JE, brewer JE. Rectilinear biphasic waveform defibrillation of out-of-hospital cardiac arrest. Prehospemerg Care. 2004;8:388-392.

[38] Gliner BE, White RD. Electrocardiographic evaluation of defibrillation shocks delivered to out-of-hospital sudden cardiac arrest patients. Resuscitation.199;41:133-144.

[39] Higgins SL, Herre JM, Epstein AE, Greer GS, Fiedman PL, Gleva ML, Porterfield JG, Chapman FW, Finkel ES, Schimdt PW. A comparison of biphasic and monophasic shocks for external defibrillation. Physio-Control Biphasic Investigators. Prehosp. Emer Care.2000;4:305-313.

[40] Steil IG, Walker RG, Nesbitt LP, Chapman FW, Cousineau D, Christenson J, Bradford P, Sookram S, berringer R, Lank P, Wells GA. BIPHASIC Trial: a randomized comparison of fixed lower versus escalating higher energy levels for defibrillation in out-of-hospital cardiac arrest. Circulation.2007;115:1511-1517

[41] MS Link, DL Atkins, Rod S. Passman et al. Part 6: Electrical Therapies: Automated External Defibrillators, Defibrillation, Cardioversion, and Pacing. 2010 American Heart Association Guidelines for Cardiopulmonary Resuscitation and Emergency Cardiovascular Care. Circulation. 2010;122:S706-S719

[42] Deale, OC, Lerman, BB. Intrathoracic current flow during transthoracic defibrillation in dogs: transcardiac current fraction. Circ Res 1990; 67:1405.

[43] Kerber RE, Kouba C, Martins J, Kelly K, Low R, Hoyt R, Ferguson D, Bailey L, Bennet P, charbonnier F. Advance prediction of transthoracic impedance in human defibrillation and cardioversion: importance of impedance in determining the success of low-energy shocks. Circulation.1984;70:303-308.

[44] Dalzell GW, Cunningham SR, Anderson J, Adgey AA. Electrode pad size, transthoracic impedance and success of external ventricular defibrillation. Am J Cardiol. 1989;64:741-744.

[45] Ewy, GA, Taren, D. Comparison of paddle electrode pastes used for defibrillation. Heart Lung 1977; 6:847.

[46] Kerber, RE, Jensen, SR, Grayzel, J, et al. Elective cardioversion: influence of paddle-electrode location and size on success rates and energy requirements. N Engl J Med 1981; 305:658.

[47] Ewy, GA, Tapen, D. Impedance to transthoracic direct current discharge: A model for testing interface material. Med Instrum 1978; 12:47.

[48] Thomas ED, Ewy GA, Dahl CF, Ewy MD. Effectiveness of direct current defibrillation: role of paddle electrode size. Am Heart J.1977;93:463-467.

[49] Dahl, CF, Ewy, GA, Warner, ED, et al. Myocardial necrosis from direct current countershock. Effect of paddle electrode size and time interval between discharges. Circulation 1974; 50:956.

[50] Atkins DL, Sirna S, ieso R, Charbonnier F, Kerber RE. Pediatricdefibrillation:importance of paddle size in determining transthoracic impedance. Pediatrics. 1988;82:914-918.

[51] Kirchhof, P, Monnig, G, Wasmer, K, et al. A trial of self-adhesive patch electrodes and hand-held paddle electrodes for external cardioversion of atrial fibrillation (MOBIPAPA). Eur Heart J 2005; 26:1292.

[52] Cummins RO, Eisenberg MS, Bergener L, Murrau JA. Sensitivity, accurancy and safety of an automatic external defibrillator. Lancet.1984;2:318-320.

[53] Dickey W, Dalzell GW, Anderson JM, Adgey AA. The accuracy of decision-making of a semi-automatic defibrillator during cardiac arrest. Eur Heart J. 1992;13:608–615.

[54] Kerber RE, Becker LB, bourland JD, Cummins RO, Hallstrom AP, Michos MB, Nichol G, Ornato JP, Et Al. Automatic external defibrillators for public access defibrillation: recommendations for specifying and reporting arrhythmia analysis algorithm performance, incorporatin new waveforms, and enhancing safety. A statement for health professionals from America Heart Association Task Force on Automatic External Defibrillation, Subcommittee on AED Safety and Efficacy. Circulation. 1997;95:1677-1682.

[55] Menegazzi JJ, Callaway CW, Sherman LD, Hostler DP, Wang HE,vFertig KC, Logue ES. Ventricular fibrillation scaling exponent can guide timing of defibrillation and other therapies. Circulation. 2004;109: 926–931.

[56] Povoas HP, Weil MH, Tang W, Bisera J, Klouche K, Barbatsis A. Predicting the success of defibrillation by electrocardiographic analysis. Resuscitation. 2002;53:77– 82.

[57] Caffrey SL, Willoughby PJ, Pepe PE, Becker LB (October 2002). "Public use of automated external defibrillators". N. Engl. J. Med. 347 (16): 1242–7.

[58] 59. Deakin C, Nolanb JP, Sunde K, Koster R. European Resuscitation Council Guidelines for Resuscitation 2010 Section 3. Electrical therapies: Automated external defibrillators, defibrillation,cardioversion and pacing.

[59] Kuisma M, Souminen P, Korpela R. Paediatric out-of-hospital cardiac arrest; epidemiology and outcame. Resuscitation.1995;30:141-150.

[60] Gurnett CA, Atkins DL. Successful use of a biphasic waveform automated external defibrillator in a high-risk child. Am J Cardiol.2000;86:1051-1053.

[61] Berg RA, Chapman FW, BERG MD, Hilwig RW, Banville I, Walker RG, Nova RC, Sherril D, Kern KB. Attenuated adult biphasic shocks compared with weight-based monophasic shocks in a swine model of prolongespediatric ventricular fibrillation. Resuscitation.2004;61:189-197.

[62] Atkins DL, Jorgenson DB.Attenuatedpediatric electrode pads for automated external defibrillator use in children. Resuscitation.2005;66:31-37.

[63] Jorgenson D, Morgan C, Snyder D, Griesse H, Solosko T, Chan K, Skarr T. Energy attenuatot for pediatric application of an automated external defibrillator in an infant.Resuscitation.2005;67:135-137.

[64] Ecker R, Rea TD, Meischke H, et al. Dispatcher assistance and automated external defibrillator performance among elders. AcadEmerg Med 2001; 8:968.

[65] Fromm RE Jr, Varon J. Automated external versus blind manual defibrillation by untrained lay rescuers. Resuscitation 1997; 33:219.

[66] Lynch B, Einspruch EL, Nichol G, et al. Effectiveness of a 30-min CPR self-instruction program for lay responders: a controlled randomized study. Resuscitation 2005; 67:31.

[67] Meischke HW, Rea T, Eisenberg MS, et al. Training seniors in the operation of an automated external defibrillator: a randomized trial comparing two training methods. Ann Emerg Med 2001; 38:216.

[68] Nichol G, Hallstrom AP, Kerber R, Moss AJ, ornate JP, plamer D, Riegel B, smith S, Weisfeldt ML. American heart Association report on the second public Access defibrillation conference, Abril 17-19, 1997.Circulation.1998;97:1309-1314.

[69] Stoddard FG. Public access defibrillation comes of age. Currents.1997;7:1-3.

[70] Watts DD. Defibrillation by basic emergency medical technicians: effect on survival. Ann Emerg Med 1995; 26:635.

[71] Auble TE, Menegazzi JJ, Paris PM. Effect of out-of-hospital defibrillation by basic life support providers on cardiac arrest mortality: a metaanalysis. Ann Emerg Med 1995; 25:642.

[72] Sweeney TA, Runge JW, Gibbs MA, et al. EMT defibrillation does not increase survival from sudden cardiac death in a two-tiered urban-suburban EMS system. Ann Emerg Med 1998; 31:234.

[73] Valenzuela TD, Kern KB, Clark LL, et al. Interruptions of chest compressions during emergency medical systems resuscitation. Circulation 2005; 112:1259.

[74] Berg RA, Hilwig RW, Kern KB, et al. Automated external defibrillation versus manual defibrillation for prolonged ventricular fibrillation: lethal delays of chest compressions before and after countershocks. Ann Emerg Med 2003; 42:458.

[75] Rea TD, Helbock M, Perry S, et al. Increasing use of cardiopulmonary resuscitation during out-of-hospital ventricular fibrillation arrest: survival implications of guideline changes. Circulation 2006; 114:2760.

[76] Bobrow BJ, Clark LL, Ewy GA, et al. Minimally interrupted cardiac resuscitation by emergency medical services for out-of-hospital cardiac arrest. JAMA 2008; 299:1158.

[77] White RD, Vukov LF, Bugliosi TF. Early defibrillation by police: initial experience with measurement of critical time intervals and patient outcome. Ann Emerg Med 1994; 23:1009.

[78] White RD, Bunch TJ, Hankins DG. Evolution of a community-wide early defibrillation programme experience over 13 years using police/fire personnel and paramedics as responders. Resuscitation 2005; 65:279.

[79] Bardy GH, Lee KL, Mark DB, et al. Home use of automated external defibrillators for sudden cardiac arrest. N Engl J Med 2008; 358:1793.

[80] Chan PS, Krumholz HM, Nichol G, et al. Delayed time to defibrillation after in-hospital cardiac arrest. N Engl J Med 2008; 358:9.

[81] Friedman FD, Dowler K, Link MS. A public access defibrillation programme in non-inpatient hospital areas. Resuscitation 2006; 69:407.

[82] Gombotz H, Weh B, Mitterndorfer W, Rehak P. In-hospital cardiac resuscitation outside the ICU by nursing staff equipped with automated external defibrillators--the first 500 cases. Resuscitation 2006; 70:416.

[83] Chan PS, Krumholz HM, Spertus JA, et al. Automated external defibrillators and survival after in-hospital cardiac arrest. JAMA 2010; 304:2129.

[84] Nichol G, Huszti E, Birnbaum A, et al. Cost-effectiveness of lay responder defibrillation for out-of-hospital cardiac arrest. Ann Emerg Med 2009; 54:226.

[85] Weisfeldt ML, Sitlani CM, Ornato JP, et al. Survival after application of automatic external defibrillators before arrival of the emergency medical system: evaluation in the resuscitation outcomes consortium population of 21 million. J Am CollCardiol 2010; 55:1713.

[86] Nichol G, Valenzuela T, Roe D, et al. Cost effectiveness of defibrillation by targeted responders in public settings. Circulation 2003; 108:697.

[87] Groeneveld PW, Kwong JL, Liu Y, et al. Cost-effectiveness of automated external defibrillators on airlines. JAMA 2001; 286:1482.

[88] Hazinski MF, Markenson D, Neish S, et al. Response to cardiac arrest and selected life-threatening medical emergencies: the medical emergency response plan for schools: A statement for healthcare providers, policymakers, school administrators, and community leaders. Circulation 2004; 109:278.

[89] Chung MK, Szymkiewicz SJ, Shao M, et al. Aggregate national experience with the wearable cardioverter-defibrillator: event rates, compliance, and survival. J Am Coll Cardiol 2010; 56:194.

[90] Klein HU, Meltendorf U, Reek S, et al. Bridging a temporary high risk of sudden arrhythmic death. Experience with the wearable cardioverter defibrillator (WCD). Pacing ClinElectrophysiol 2010; 33:353.

[91] Li Y, Bisera J, Tang W, Weil MH. Automated detection of ventricular fibrillation to guide cardiopulmonary resuscitation. CritPathwCardiol 2007; 6:131.

[92] Berger RD, Palazzolo J, Halperin H. Rhythm discrimination during uninterrupted CPR using motion artifact reduction system. Resuscitation 2007; 75:145.

Section 2

Principals of Internal Cardiac Defibrillation

Chapter 2

Defibrillation and Cardiac Geometry

Dan Blendea, Razvan Dadu and Craig A. McPherson

Additional information is available at the end of the chapter

http://dx.doi.org/10.5772/55120

1. Introduction

Although ICD therapy is an efficient and reliable therapeutic method, internal defibrillation is a traumatic experience; moreover and there is accumulating evidence that internal defibrillation, especially with high defibrillation energy, may adversely affect cardiac function and even patient prognosis [1, 2]. Therefore, considerable research efforts have been focused on better defining defibrillation mechanisms, particularly aiming at and improving defibrillation efficacy and in order to reduce lowering defibrillation energy requirements.

Recent developments in cardiac simulation have been used to create more accurate defibrillation models. The chapter tries to focus on the importance of geometry in the different defibrillation models, and explores potential applications of these models to improve the transvenous defibrillation systems, and the more recently developed extracardiac ICDs.

2. Geometry and pathogenesis of ventricular fibrillation

The exact mechanism of ventricular fibrillation (VF) is still unknown. One of the most accepted hypotheses is that during VF, synchronous contraction of the muscle is disrupted by fast, vortex-like, rotating waves of electrical activity named rotors.[3-6]. The spiral wave rotates about an organizing center, or core, which is thought to be an unexcited but excitable medium that defines the primary dynamic characteristics of the wave. At the core of the vortex is a line of phase singularities (i.e. a region where the phase is undefined) named filament. It seems that, at least in the initial phases, a relatively stable circuit, called the mother rotor, maintains VF.[7] Zaitsev et al[7] used the term domain to define a region in which all of the tissue has the same peak frequency in the VF power spectrum.[8] Optical recordings during VF found that a single domain of highest peak frequency was present, named the dominant domain, and was surrounded by domains of lower peak frequencies. Some wavefronts that arouse in the dominant domain propagate into domains with lower peak frequencies, and others block at the boundary between domains.[9] These findings suggest that that VF is maintained by a single, stationary, stable reentrant circuit, i.e., the mother rotor, in the dominant domain, which has the shortest refractory period from which activations propagate into the more slowly activating domains with longer refractory periods. Nanthakumar et al [10] demonstrated reentrant wavefronts in human VF, providing a direct demonstration of phase singularities, wavebreaks and rotor formation in severely diseased, explanted human hearts.[11] Importantly, they found also wavefronts as large as the entire vertical length of the optical field, which suggested a high degree of organization.[10] Findings from simultaneous epicardial and endocardial multielectrode mapping in patients with cardiomyopathy [12] suggested that during induced VF episodes, stable reentrant wavefronts occur in the endocardium and the epicardium. The same authors demonstrated a stable source in the endocardium, with a highly organized pattern in the local electrogram and a simultaneous and disorganized pattern in the epicardium, consistent with the hypothesis of 3-dimensional scroll waves.[12] Thus, the short-lived rotors on the epicardial and/or endocardial surfaces are thought to be manifestations of a scroll wave organized along the fiber orientation within the wall. Massé et al also observed variable block patterns in wavefront transmission, resulting in disorganized activity and wavefront fragmentation.[12] Rotors may exist alone as stationary high-frequency mother rotors that generate wavefronts that fractionate and disorganize in its periphery. They may also manifest as drifting rotors or even as rotors that rapidly die off leaving multiple offspring wavelets that originate new short-lived rotors and new wavelets.[11]

3. Rotors and heart geometry

Rotors are common to many biological, chemical and physical excitable media and their dynamics have been researched intensively. The specific anatomical structure of the cardiac chambers is likely to be a crucial factor in determining the fibrillatory behavior. The heterogeneity of the ventricular anatomy is likely to play an important role in rotor dynamics. For example, the thicker left ventricular wall may manifest the complex dynamics of 3-dimensional scroll waves much more readily than the thinner right ventricle and the atrial walls. There is a left-to-right gradient of dominant frequencies, suggesting that the left heart may be playing the leading role in maintaining fibrillation. [11] Kim et al. suggested that sink-to-source mismatch between areas with different thickness in the ventricle may serve to anchor rotors [13] and these rotors may span the thickness of the ventricular wall. For instance, the papillary muscles in the LV may help to stabilize rotors.[11,14]

A thickness threshold is sought at which complex and changing short-period wave behavior abruptly becomes more organized into simple drifting spiral waves of slightly longer period. [15 16] Such a threshold was indeed found in canine ventricles and bears the same relation to rotor period and representing about $1/\pi$ times the distance a spiral wave propagates during one rotation period.[16] This distance is the nominal diameter of the rotor, the source of the reentrant activation front. In three dimensions, this source is not, as in two dimensions, a small elliptical disk but a filament.[16] If the myocardial tissue is thick enough to admit a vortex filament lying on its side, the rotor can move more freely, fragment, and close in rings.[16] In numerical experiments with uniformly anisotropic and perfectly continuous and homogeneous three-dimensional excitable media, such vortex filaments spontaneously lash about unless confined to a layer thinner than about a rotor diameter.[16] Apart from reasonably steady rotation, their motion is apparently irregular. It seems that there is a thickness threshold of about one rotor diameter (3 to 10 mm, depending on fiber orientation) that complements the known area threshold for creating and sustaining a rotor (3 mm by 3 or 10 mm perpendicular to thickness, depending on fiber orientation). Together, they constitute a compact critical volume of 3 mm by 3 mm by 10 mm (about 0.1 g of tissue) beyond which reentrant tachycardia (monomorphic or polymorphic) can spontaneously become more complex (fibrillation).[16] Another finding suggesting role of tissue thickness for development of ventricular fibrillation is the observation that rotors in situ have a longer period in thinner (and more epicardial) layers.[17] Another possible contributor to the thickness effect arises from the conspicuous rotation of fiber orientation from epicardium to endocardium. It has been suggested that twist renders vortex filaments unstable.[18] There is a suggestion that thicker myocardium, bearing less twist per unit distance, would be less liable to such instabilities. The thinner right ventricular free wall is capable of supporting spiral waves more stably, and the thicker left ventricular wall more often degenerates to fibrillation. [16,19]

An interesting analysis that gives more insight into the pathogenesis of rotor is a correlation of body size, heart weight, ventricular surface area, and wall thickness in different mammalians against the minimum safely sustainable sinus rhythm interval over different species. This analysis assumes that the rotor dynamics is the same in the ventricular myocardium of different mammalian species.[16] Data from mammals including rats, guinea pigs, and man shows that rotors thus turn out to lie on the phylogenetic trend line near the transition from normal hearts that spontaneously defibrillate to normal hearts capable of sustained fibrillation. It seems that ventricles cannot stably beat faster than the rotor period unless they are too small to accommodate a rotor. Individuals susceptible to death by ventricular fibrillation have sufficient ventricular surface dimensions to accommodate a rotor pair (I to 2 cm in longitudinal fiber direction) and have a wall thickness sufficient to accommodate a vortex filament of one rotor diameter [transverse to fibers, with anisotropically reduced electrical scale, about (1 cm)/ 3 = 3 to 4 mm.[16] Structural remodeling has been shown to interfere with rotor behavior. With regards to the ventricles, it has been shown experimentally that the dynamics of VF in the presence of heart failure are different from those in the normal heart. Heart failure remodeling decreases VF rate and increases VF organization.[11]

4. Geometry and defibrillation

The only clinically effective method for eliminating vortices in the heart is the delivery of a high-energy electric shock that depolarizes and also hyperpolarizes the tissue with a voltage gradient of about 5 V/cm.[6] In the bidomain representation, the voltage in cardiac tissue is the potential drop between the intracellular and extracellular medium. Theory predicts [20] that, in the presence of an electric field, discontinuities in tissue conductivity, such as blood vessels, changes in fiber direction, fatty tissue and intercellular clefts, induce a redistribution of intracellular and extracellular currents that can locally hyperpolarize or depolarize the cells. At the depolarization threshold, an excitation wave is emitted.[6,20,21] Conceptually, defibrillation can be considered to be a two-step process. Firstly, the applied shock drives currents that traverse the myocardium and cause complex polarization changes in transmembrane potential distribution. Secondly, post-shock active membrane reactions are invoked that eventually result either in termination of ventricular fibrillation in the case of shock success, or in reinitiation of fibrillatory activity in the case of shock failure.[22]

Over a decade ago, bidomain simulations[23] followed by optical mapping studies [24,25] demonstrated that the membrane response in the vicinity of a strong unipolar stimulus involved simultaneous occurrence of positive (depolarizing) and negative (hyperpolarizing) effects in close proximity. This finding of 'virtual electrodes' was in contrast with the established view [26] that tissue responses should only be depolarizing (hyperpolarizing) if the stimulus was cathodal (anodal).[27] Essentially, the virtual electrode polarization (VEP) theory states that adjacent areas of opposite polarizations exist around the tip of the pacing electrode.[28] Sepulveda et al. [23] showed that the region depolarized (excited) by a strong stimulus has a dog-bone shape, with its long axis perpendicular to the direction of the myocardial fibers. Regions of hyperpolarization (called virtual anodes) exist adjacent to the electrode along the fiber direction. A virtual anode is an example of a virtual electrode. Many researchers have observed these regions of depolarization and hyperpolarization experimentally. [25,29] Depolarization can excite a cell and conversely, hyperpolarization can de-excite a cell. The cellular response to shock-induced VEP depends on the strength and polarity of the shock, as well as on the electrophysiological state of the cell at the time of shock delivery. Positive VEP can result in regenerative depolarization in regions where tissue is at or near diastole; such activation is termed 'make' because it takes place at the onset (make) of the shock. A strong negative VEP can completely abolish the action potential (i.e. regenerative repolarization), thus creating post-shock excitable gaps in the virtual anode regions. The close proximity of a de-excited region and a virtual cathode has been shown, in both modelling studies and optical mapping experiments,[25] to result in an excitation at shock end (termed 'break' excitation, i.e. at the break of the shock). The virtual cathode serves as an electrical stimulus eliciting a regenerative depolarization and a propagating wave in the newly created excitable gap.[27] For a defibrillation shock to succeed, it must extinguish existing VF activations throughout the myocardium (or in a critical mass of it), as well as not initiate new fibrillatory wavefronts.[27] A shock succeeds in extinguishing fibrillatory wavefronts and not initiating new re-entry if make/break excitations manage to traverse the shock-induced excitable gaps before the rest of the myocardium recovers from shock-induced depolarization.[27] Defibrillation failure has been explained by one (or both) of the following mechanisms: (I) the shock fails to extinguish all or a sufficient amount of fibrillatory electrical activity and (2) newly created shock-induced wavebreaks by near-threshold stimulating fields occurring at existing excitable gaps.[30]

Detailed analysis of VEP etiology demonstrated that both applied field [24] and tissue structure are major determinants of the shape, location, polarity and intensity of the shock-induced polarization.[24,27] The cellular response to shock-induced VEP depends on the strength and polarity of the shock, as well as on the electrophysiological state of the cell at the time of shock delivery.[27] There is a relationship between the response of the tissue to an electric field and the spatial distribution of heterogeneities in the scale-free coronary vascular structure. In response to a pulsed electric field, these heterogeneities serve as nucleation sites for the generation of intramural electrical waves that can generate tissue depolarization. These intramural wave sources permit targeting of electrical turbulence near the cores of the vortices of electrical activity that drive complex fibrillatory dynamics. Simultaneous and direct access to multiple vortex cores results in rapid synchronization of cardiac tissue and therefore, efficient termination of fibrillation. Using this control strategy, Luther et al. demonstrated low-energy termination of fibrillation in vivo. Their results give new insights into the mechanisms and dynamics underlying the control of spatio-temporal chaos in heterogeneous excitable media and provide new research perspectives towards alternative, life-saving low-energy defibrillation techniques.[6]

5. Geometry and lead positioning for cardiac defibrillation

Most models used to describe defibrillation view the myocardial mass as an isotropic conductive domain and use the critical mass hypothesis to define successful defibrillation. According to this hypothesis the success of a defibrillation shock depends on rendering a critical mass of the myocardium inexcitable, such that fibrillation wavefronts have no myocardium to depolarize and propagate through.[19] It has been found that raising the extracellular potential gradient above a critical level renders myocardium refractory.[31] Frazier et al.[32] have found the critical level of potential gradient to be close to 5 V/cm, and a commonly accepted value for critical myocardial mass is 95%. [33]

In a recent study Yang et al. examined the effect of coil position on active-can single-coil ICD defibrillation efficacy by using a finite difference thoracic model which incorporated realistic geometries and conductive inhomogeneities of human thoracic tissues. [34] Four electrode configurations with the coil placed, respectively, in the right ventricular (RV) apex, in the middle of RV cavity, along the free wall in RV, or along the septal wall in RV, were simulated and their defibrillation efficacies were evaluated based on a set of metrics including voltage defibrillation threshold (VDFT) and current defibrillation threshold. It was found that the optimal electrode configuration is to position the coil in the middle of the RV cavity.

The RV cavity-to-can configuration had more endocardium exposed to the more uniform and relatively high voltage gradient fields. Other configurations exposed only endocardic surfaces near the electrodes to high voltage gradient fields and the voltage gradient drops more quickly in myocardial tissue as its resistivity value is one-third larger than blood's.

Aguel et al[35] used a high-resolution finite element model of a human torso that includes the fiber architecture of the ventricular myocardium to find the role of lead positioning in a transvenous lead-to-can defibrillation electrode system. They found that, among single lead systems, posterior positioning of leads in the right ventricle lowers VDFTs. Furthermore, a septal location of leads resulted in lower VDFTs than free-wall positioning. Increasing the number of leads, and thus the effective lead surface area in the right ventricle also resulted in lower VDFTs. However, the lead configuration that resulted in the lowest VDFTs is a combination of mid-cavity right ventricle lead and a mid-cavity left ventricle lead.

Since the shape of the myocardial mass–voltage gradient curve is determined entirely by the geometry of the model and the lead design,[35] an improvement in defibrillation efficacy may be achieved by adjustment of the defibrillation lead surface and position, as this allows a more even distribution of the voltage gradient field over a wider surface of the myocardium.[36] Although centering the coils inside the heart chambers is probably not feasible with the current leads, positioning the coil in the middle of the RV cavity functioned equivalently in this sense as it had almost the entire RV endocardial surface exposed to a relatively evenly distributed voltage gradient field considering blood's resistivity is significantly less than the resistivity value of myocardium.

Current density distribution is another important parameter to use in evaluating the efficacy of defibrillation. The cross-sectional current density distribution showed that in the full tissue model skeletal muscle provided an alternative pathway for the current flow. By calculating the current flowing through various regions in the cross-sections it was found that more than 25% of the total current passing through the cross-sections flowed through the skeletal muscle around the outer boundary of the thorax, independent of electrode configuration. On average, 10% of the current was shunted through the relatively high resistivity fat on the outer boundaries of the thorax and another 10% was shunted though the left lung. This suggests that the amount of skeletal muscle, fat and lungs impact the amount of current reaching the heart. This finding is consistent with the results reported by Geddes et al.[37] that indicates body size or shape has a significant influence on the amount of current required for successful defibrillation, though it was based on studies of transthoracic ventricular defibrillation. Examining the current flowing through the heart in the cross-sections on the average, less than 10% of the current flowed through the myocardium, and a major portion of the current flowing through the heart region was shunted through the blood chambers.[34] In a simplified view, the current from the electrode in the RV can propagate up through the blood chambers to the base of the heart, great vessels, and lung to the can, or out through the myocardial wall to the skeletal muscle and up to the can. Both paths are used, but as the ventricles become more enlarged as in patients with advanced heart failure, the low resistivity blood shifts more current up through the base of the heart and away from the skeletal muscle.[34] This would suggest that the large heart chambers of patients in heart failure, or with an enlarged heart, would tend to shunt the current away from the myocardial tissue in the middle regions of the heart, thus resulting in the need for higher defibrillation currents.[34]

5.1. Clinical aspects of right ventricular lead positioning for defibrillation

Until relatively recently lead placement in the RV apex has been the standard of care for patients requiring pacemaker or defibrillator lead placement (Figure 1).[38]

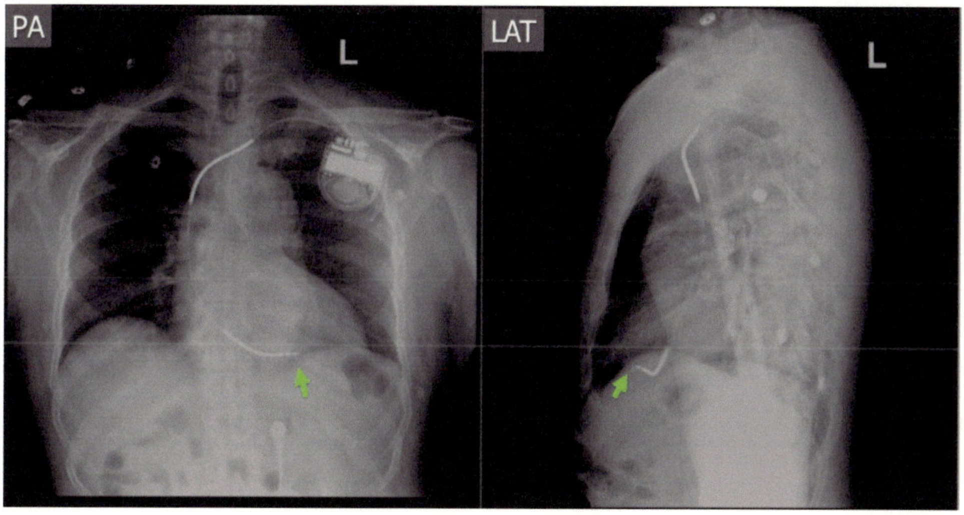

Figure 1. Single chamber dual coil ICD system with the lead placed in the apex of the right ventricle (arrow). Postero-anterior (PA) and lateral (LAT) radiographic views.

It was advised to place the RV coil towards the apex to reduce the DFTs, mainly driven by data obtained before the active can configurations were introduced.[38] Without the hot can pulling current toward the apex, it was important to have the RV coil tip deep in the apex. Otherwise, the current would tend to follow the blood pool back to the SVC coil, shunting the defibrillation energy away from the LV myocardium and raising the VDFT. [38] With a chest electrode ("hot can") in place, the RV apical position is not as critical because current is pulled directed from whatever position in the RV that the coil resides, through the apex to the pectoralis major muscle and to the hot can, thereby including the LV myocardium in the wave front's path.[39] Actually with a hot can, and with no SVC coil, the apical position was shown to be inferior in terms of DFTs.[34] If a hot can and an SVC coil are used the data available seems to suggest a slight advantage for the RV apex position. Clinical studies comparing the DFT for an RV coil tip in the apex versus in the right ventricular outflow tract using biphasic waveforms and a hot can showed that the mean benefit of an apical position was approximately 10% DFT reduction.[38,40,41] This relatively small benefit must be weighed against the increased risk of perforation associated with apical lead positioning.[38,42] Based on the current data the best compromise position of the RV coil tip seems to be along the septum midway (Figure 2) between the apex and RVOT (Figure 3).

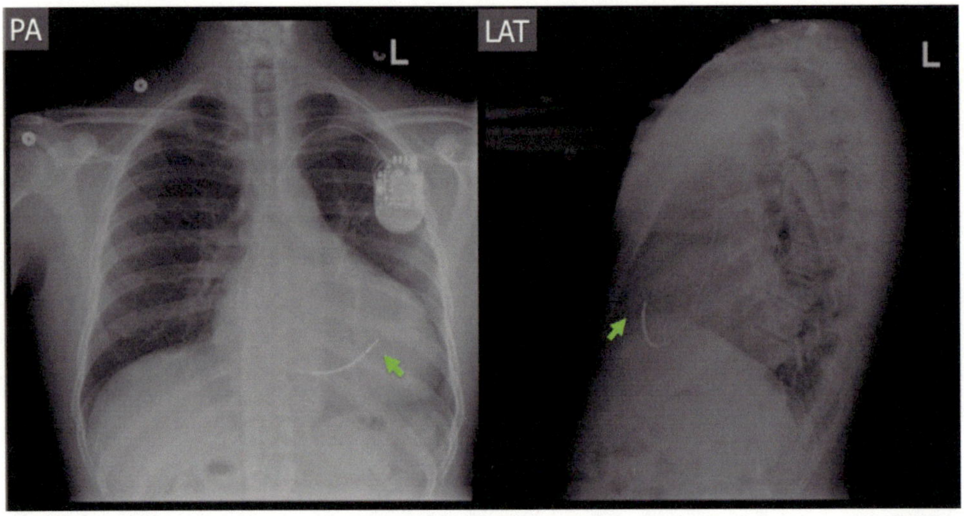

Figure 2. Single-chamber single-coil ICD system with the lead placed in a mid-septal location (arrow). Postero-anterior (PA) and lateral (LAT) radiographic views.

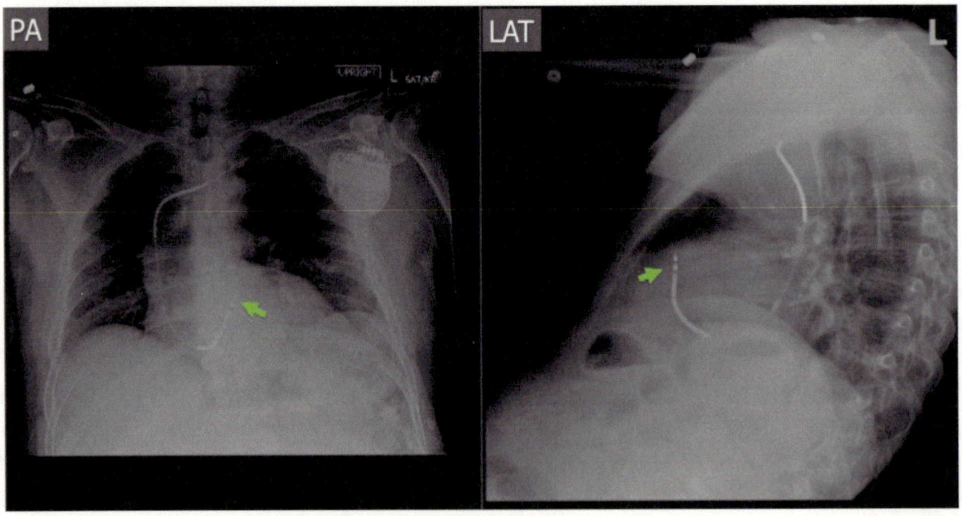

Figure 3. Single-chamber dual-coil ICD system with the lead placed at the base of the right ventricular outflow tract (arrow). Postero-anterior (PA) and lateral (LAT) radiographic views.

If the SVC coil is used, (given the lower DFTs for the mid-septal/RVOT position) an apical or apical-septal position may be considered (Figure 1). If the SVC coil is not used, the mid-septal location (Figure 2) appears to give lower DFTs than the apical tip location according to a modeling study.[34,38]

The effect of waveform polarity has been studied using both monophasic and biphasic waveforms, and the available data shows 15-20% DFT mean reduction when an anodal RV coil configuration is being used. [38,43] These results are predicted by the virtual electrode hypothesis of defibrillation[44] that predicts that post-shock virtual electrodes launch new wavefronts toward the anode.[38] A right ventricular cathode produces expanding, pro-arrhythmic wavefronts, whereas a right ventricular anode produces collapsing, self-extinguishing wavefronts. [38] An additional beneficial effect of anodal RV shocks may be to increase the homogeneity of membrane time constants in comparison with cathodal shocks.[38,45]

Another element of lead technology that can affect the efficiency of a defibrillation system is the SVC coil. Studies on patients with active-can lead configurations suggest that the addition of the SVC coil decreases the DFT and reduces impedance. With an apically placed RV coil and a prepectoral hot can, major current flow is to the pectoralis major and to the ICD can. Minimal current flows to the posterior base. The addition of an SVC coil directs some current vertically and toward the posterior.

There are several detrimental effects from the use of the SVC coil, especially for a coil placed in the right atrium. The low SVC coil diverts current from the apex and LV free wall because the RV and atrial blood pool provide a lower resistance path. In addition, a low cathodal SVC coil could launch wavefronts into basal RV. And, additionally, the extraction of a dual-coil lead is much more challenging because the adherences that can form between the SVC coil and the venous wall.[38]

A recent study analyzed comparatively the DFTs for active and inactive SVC coils.[46] The results depended on the single coil impedance. If the single coil impedance was >58Ω, then an active SVC coil almost always lowered the DFT. If the single coil impedance was already in the normal range (<58 Ω), then the effect of the SVC coil was split.[38] Half of patients had a lower DFT and half had a higher DFT. Interestingly, if the SVC coil was active, its position was important: an SVC coil in the SVC/right atrial junction increased the DFT, and an SVC coil placed in the SVC/ innominate junction decreased the DFT.[46]

6. Electrode configurations for subcutaneous ICDs

Total subcutaneous implantable subcutaneous defibrillators (S-ICDs) have been developed as alternative ICD strategies allowing more widespread application of ICD therapy for the primary prevention of sudden death. The optimal device and electrode configurations for S-ICDs are not well known. Image-based defibrillation finite element models have been used to predict the myocardial electric field generated during defibrillation shocks in a variety of subcutaneous electrode positions, in order to determine factors affecting optimal lead positions for subcutaneous ICDs (S-ICD), and ultimately to improve the efficacy of these defibrillation systems.

Jolley et al.[47] used image-based finite element models (FEM) to predict the myocardial electric field generated during defibrillation shocks (pseudo-DFT) in a wide variety of subcutaneous electrode positions to determine factors affecting optimal lead positions for subcutaneous implantable cardioverter-defibrillators (S-ICD). An image-based FEM of an adult man was used to predict pseudo-DFTs across a wide range of technically feasible S-ICD electrode placements. Generator location, lead location, length, geometry and orientation, and spatial relation of electrodes to ventricular mass were systematically varied. Best electrode configurations were determined, and spatial factors contributing to low pseudo-DFTs were identified using regression and general linear models.[47] One previously published and validated S-ICD configuration[48] was selected as the base case for normalization of the predicted DFTs of all tested configurations. This is the system proposed by Lieberman et al[48], which uses a low, medial pectoral position of an active generator and a 25-cm posterolateral electrode extending around the back of the left thorax between the 6th and 10th intercostal space, extending the tip as close to the spine as possible.

The study by Jolley and colleagues revealed that a wide variety of conceivable electrode orientations, some of them quite unusual and not previously reported, were predicted to be as effective or more effective than the base case (pseudo-DFT ratio <=1).[47] Univariate modeling results suggested that a variety of anatomical factors affecting the geometry of system configuration influenced pseudo-DFT. Placement of the generator in the parasternal position was more efficient than more lateral and remote positions (mid-clavicular, anterior-axillary, abdominal). Anterolateral and posterior electrode positions were better than para-sternal, and anterolateral better than anterior. Right-sided generators were more efficient than left-sided generators, whereas the converse was true for electrode laterality. Although some of these alternatives represent simple modifications of the previously proposed system, many involve changes in lead design and implant technique that are substantial; in particular, the contralateral placement of generator and lead.

Multivariate modeling using linear regression models showed that favorable alignment of shock vector with ventricular myocardium, increased lead length, can horizontal position, contralateral lead-generator position, and distance of can from the heart independently predicted pseudo-DFTs. The relative positions of the generator, the lead(s), and the ventricular myocardium accounted for nearly half of the predicted variability in the pseudo-DFT. This reflects the intuitive observation that electrodes should be positioned to place the heart as nearly between them as possible. This multivariate analysis revealed important principles that may guide the design of subcutaneous ICDs. Placement of the electrodes to align the inter-electrode shock vector as closely as possible to the center of mass of the ventricular myocar-dium, and use of longer electrode coil lengths are associated with lower DFTs and account for the majority of variability of this parameter. Manipulation of electrode length contributed almost 25% of the variability in pseudo-DFTs, with decreases in pseudo-DFTs predicted with extension of coil length from 5 to 10 cm and longer. Neither of these factors has previously been quantified for subcutaneous electrode placement and may prove useful in determining optimal orientations. Notably, although electrode arrays were often identified as useful in many efficient configurations, the use of an array was generally not necessarily more efficient than a single electrode of equal length similarly positioned. This finding implies both for S-

http://dx.doi.org/10.5772/55120

ICD design and for current subcutaneous arrays used to augment transvenous systems with unacceptably high DFTs that a simple, single-electrode system is likely to offer as much benefit as an array, which is more difficult to implant and may be more prone to failure.

Author details

Dan Blendea[1], Razvan Dadu[2] and Craig A. McPherson[2]

1 Massachusetts General Hospital - Harvard Medical School, USA

2 Bridgeport Hospital – Yale University School of Medicine, USA

References

[1] Poole, J. E, Johnson, G. W, Hellkamp, A. S, et al. Prognostic importance of defibrillator shocks in patients with heart failure. N Engl J Med (2008)., 359, 1009-17.

[2] Blendea, D, Blendea, M, Banker, J, & Mcpherson, C. A. Troponin T elevation after implanted defibrillator discharge predicts survival. Heart (2009)., 95, 1153-8.

[3] Davidenko, J. M, Pertsov, A. V, Salomonsz, R, Baxter, W, & Jalife, J. Stationary and drifting spiral waves of excitation in isolated cardiac muscle. Nature (1992)., 355, 349-51.

[4] Gray, R. A, Pertsov, A. M, & Jalife, J. Spatial and temporal organization during cardiac fibrillation. Nature (1998)., 392, 75-8.

[5] Witkowski, F. X, Leon, L. J, Penkoske, P. A, et al. Spatiotemporal evolution of ventricular fibrillation. Nature (1998)., 392, 78-82.

[6] Luther, S, Fenton, F. H, Kornreich, B. G, et al. Low-energy control of electrical turbulence in the heart. Nature (2011)., 475, 235-9.

[7] Zaitsev, A. V, Berenfeld, O, Mironov, S. F, Jalife, J, & Pertsov, A. M. Distribution of excitation frequencies on the epicardial and endocardial surfaces of fibrillating ventricular wall of the sheep heart. Circ Res (2000)., 86, 408-17.

[8] Tabereaux, P. B, Dosdall, D. J, & Ideker, R. E. Mechanisms of VF maintenance: wandering wavelets, mother rotors, or foci. Heart Rhythm (2009)., 6, 405-15.

[9] Samie, F. H, Berenfeld, O, Anumonwo, J, et al. Rectification of the background potassium current: a determinant of rotor dynamics in ventricular fibrillation. Circ Res (2001)., 89, 1216-23.

[10] Nanthakumar, K, Jalife, J, Masse, S, et al. Optical mapping of Langendorff-perfused human hearts: establishing a model for the study of ventricular fibrillation in humans. Am J Physiol Heart Circ Physiol (2007). H, 875-80.

[11] Vaquero, M, Calvo, D, & Jalife, J. Cardiac fibrillation: from ion channels to rotors in the human heart. Heart Rhythm (2008). , 5, 872-9.

[12] Masse, S, Downar, E, Chauhan, V, Sevaptsidis, E, & Nanthakumar, K. Ventricular fibrillation in myopathic human hearts: mechanistic insights from in vivo global endocardial and epicardial mapping. Am J Physiol Heart Circ Physiol (2007). H, 2589-97.

[13] Kim, Y. H, Yashima, M, Wu, T. J, Doshi, R, Chen, P. S, & Karagueuzian, H. S. Mechanism of procainamide-induced prevention of spontaneous wave break during ventricular fibrillation. Insight into the maintenance of fibrillation wave fronts. Circulation (1999). , 100, 666-74.

[14] Wu, T. J, Lin, S. F, Baher, A, et al. Mother rotors and the mechanisms of D600-induced type 2 ventricular fibrillation. Circulation (2004). , 110, 2110-8.

[15] Winfree, A. T. Scroll-shaped waves of chemical activity in three dimensions. Science (1973). , 181, 937-9.

[16] Winfree, A. T. Electrical turbulence in three-dimensional heart muscle. Science (1994). , 266, 1003-6.

[17] Kavanagh, K. M, Kabas, J. S, Rollins, D. L, Melnick, S. B, Smith, W. M, & Ideker, R. E. High-current stimuli to the spared epicardium of a large infarct induce ventricular tachycardia. Circulation (1992). , 85, 680-98.

[18] Panfilov, A. V, & Keener, J. P. Generation of reentry in anisotropic myocardium. J Cardiovasc Electrophysiol (1993). , 4, 412-21.

[19] Zipes, D. P, Fischer, J, & King, R. M. Nicoll Ad, Jolly WW. Termination of ventricular fibrillation in dogs by depolarizing a critical amount of myocardium. Am J Cardiol (1975). , 36, 37-44.

[20] Plonsey, R. The nature of sources of bioelectric and biomagnetic fields. Biophys J (1982). , 39, 309-12.

[21] Fast, V. G, Rohr, S, Gillis, A. M, & Kleber, A. G. Activation of cardiac tissue by extracellular electrical shocks: formation of'secondary sources' at intercellular clefts in monolayers of cultured myocytes. Circ Res (1998). , 82, 375-85.

[22] Trayanova, N, Constantino, J, Ashihara, T, & Plank, G. Modeling defibrillation of the heart: approaches and insights. IEEE Rev Biomed Eng (2011). , 4, 89-102.

[23] Sepulveda, N. G, Roth, B. J, & Wikswo, J. P. Jr. Current injection into a two-dimensional anisotropic bidomain. Biophys J (1989). , 55, 987-99.

[24] Knisley, S. B, Trayanova, N, & Aguel, F. Roles of electric field and fiber structure in cardiac electric stimulation. Biophys J (1999). , 77, 1404-17.

[25] Wikswo, J. P. Jr., Lin SF, Abbas RA. Virtual electrodes in cardiac tissue: a common mechanism for anodal and cathodal stimulation. Biophys J (1995). , 69, 2195-210.

[26] Hodgkin, A. L, & Rushton, W. A. The electrical constants of a crustacean nerve fibre. Proc R Soc Med (1946). , 134, 444-79.

[27] Trayanova, N. Defibrillation of the heart: insights into mechanisms from modelling studies. Exp Physiol (2006). , 91, 323-37.

[28] Sambelashvili, A. T, Nikolski, V. P, & Efimov, I. R. Virtual electrode theory explains pacing threshold increase caused by cardiac tissue damage. Am J Physiol Heart Circ Physiol (2004). H, 2183-94.

[29] Knisley, S. B, Hill, B. C, & Ideker, R. E. Virtual electrode effects in myocardial fibers. Biophys J (1994). , 66, 719-28.

[30] Efimov, I. R, Gray, R. A, & Roth, B. J. Virtual electrodes and deexcitation: new insights into fibrillation induction and defibrillation. J Cardiovasc Electrophysiol (2000). , 11, 339-53.

[31] Lepeschkin, E, Jones, J. L, Rush, S, & Jones, R. E. Local potential gradients as a unifying measure for thresholds of stimulation, standstill, tachyarrhythmia and fibrillation appearing after strong capacitor discharges. Adv Cardiol (1978). , 21, 268-78.

[32] Frazier, D. W, Wolf, P. D, Wharton, J. M, Tang, A. S, Smith, W. M, & Ideker, R. E. Stimulus-induced critical point. Mechanism for electrical initiation of reentry in normal canine myocardium. J Clin Invest (1989). , 83, 1039-52.

[33] Ideker, R. E, Wolf, P. D, Alferness, C, Krassowska, W, & Smith, W. M. Current concepts for selecting the location, size and shape of defibrillation electrodes. Pacing Clin Electrophysiol (1991). , 14, 227-40.

[34] Yang, F, & Patterson, R. Optimal transvenous coil position on active-can single-coil ICD defibrillation efficacy: a simulation study. Ann Biomed Eng (2008). , 36, 1659-67.

[35] Aguel, F, Eason, J. C, Trayanova, N. A, Siekas, G, & Fishler, M. G. Impact of transvenous lead position on active-can ICD defibrillation: a computer simulation study. Pacing Clin Electrophysiol (1999). , 22, 158-64.

[36] Witkowski, F. X, Penkoske, P. A, & Plonsey, R. Mechanism of cardiac defibrillation in open-chest dogs with unipolar DC-coupled simultaneous activation and shock potential recordings. Circulation (1990). , 82, 244-60.

[37] Geddes, L. A, Tacker, W. A, Rosborough, J. P, Moore, A. G, & Cabler, P. S. Electrical dose for ventricular defibrillation of large and small animals using precordial electrodes. J Clin Invest (1974). , 53, 310-9.

[38] Kroll, M. W, & Schwab, J. O. Achieving low defibrillation thresholds at implant: pharmacological influences, RV coil polarity and position, SVC coil usage and positioning, pulse width settings, and the azygous vein. Fundam Clin Pharmacol (2010)., 24, 561-73.

[39] Usui, M, & Walcott, G. P. KenKnight BH, et al. Influence of malpositioned transvenous leads on defibrillation efficacy with and without a subcutaneous array electrode. Pacing Clin Electrophysiol (1995)., 18, 2008-16.

[40] Crossley, G. H, Boyce, K, Roelke, M, et al. A prospective randomized trial of defibrillation thresholds from the right ventricular outflow tract and the right ventricular apex. Pacing Clin Electrophysiol (2009)., 32, 166-71.

[41] Mollerus, M, Lipinski, M, & Munger, T. A randomized comparison of defibrillation thresholds in the right ventricular outflow tract versus right ventricular apex. J Interv Card Electrophysiol (2008)., 22, 221-5.

[42] Turakhia, M, Prasad, M, Olgin, J, et al. Rates and severity of perforation from implantable cardioverter-defibrillator leads: a 4-year study. J Interv Card Electrophysiol (2009)., 24, 47-52.

[43] Swerdlow, C. D, Davie, S, Ahern, T, & Chen, P. S. Comparative reproducibility of defibrillation threshold and upper limit of vulnerability. Pacing Clin Electrophysiol (1996)., 19, 2103-11.

[44] Efimov, I. R, Cheng, Y, Yamanouchi, Y, & Tchou, P. J. Direct evidence of the role of virtual electrode-induced phase singularity in success and failure of defibrillation. J Cardiovasc Electrophysiol (2000)., 11, 861-8.

[45] Kroll, M. W. A minimal model of the single capacitor biphasic defibrillation waveform. Pacing Clin Electrophysiol (1994)., 17, 1782-92.

[46] Gold, M, Val-mejias, J, Leman, R. B, et al. Optimization of superior vena cava coil position and usage for transvenous defibrillation. Heart Rhythm (2008)., 5, 394-9.

[47] Jolley, M, Stinstra, J, Tate, J, et al. Finite element modeling of subcutaneous implantable defibrillator electrodes in an adult torso. Heart Rhythm (2010)., 7, 692-8.

[48] Lieberman, R, Havel, W. J, Rashba, E, Degroot, P. J, Stromberg, K, & Shorofsky, S. R. Acute defibrillation performance of a novel, non-transvenous shock pathway in adult ICD indicated patients. Heart Rhythm (2008)., 5, 28-34.

Section 3

Worth Knowing About Indication, Long-Term Benefit, Challenges, and Monitoring of ICD Therapy

Chapter 3

Sudden Death in Ischemic Heart Disease

Elisabete Martins

Additional information is available at the end of the chapter

http://dx.doi.org/10.5772/52661

1. Introduction

Sudden cardiac death (SCD) is defined by the death from unexpected circulatory arrest, usually due to a cardiac arrhythmia occurring within one hour of the onset of symptoms [1].

It is a major health problem worldwide, with a prevalence estimated in the range of 300 000 to 350 000 cases per year in the United States [2]. Event rates in Europe are similar to those in United States [3].

Coronary heart disease (CHD) is the leading cause of SCD explaining approximately 80% of cases [4]; cardiomyopathies and primary electrical abnormalities account for most of the remainder. Approximately 50% to 70% of these deaths are related to ventricular tachyarrhythmias (ventricular fibrillation/ tachycardia) [5].

Available medical therapies, such as beta-blockers [6] or anthiarrhytmic drugs including amiodarone, failed to abolish the occurrence of SCD after a myocardial infarction (MI) [7], [8].

Implantable cardioverter defibrillators (ICD) are devices currently available capable of abort life-threatening ventricular tachyarrhythmias and therefore prevent SCD.

Although it is not possible to prevent all cases of SCD in the general population, the main issue is the identification of individuals at increased risk that may benefit from ICD implantation.

The highest risk of SCD in various heart diseases, either genetic or acquired, is related with the previous occurrence of ventricular arrhythmias [9].In secondary prevention, predominantly three randomized clinical trials have established the criteria for ICD implantation.

The antiarrhythmics versus Implantable Defibrillators (AVID) trial showed mortality reduction with ICD among survivors of ventricular fibrillation or sustained ventricular tachycardia causing severe symptoms [10]. The Canadian Implantable Defibrillator Study (CIDS) trial showed a 20% relative risk reduction in mortality with ICD therapy compared to amiodarone [11], although not statistically significant. The Cardiac Arrest Study Hamburg (CASH) trial confirm, though not with a statistical level of significance, the beneficial role of ICD therapy in the treatment of cardiac arrest survivors during long-term follow-up [12].A meta-analysis of these trials showed a 28% reduction in mortality due predominantly to a reduction in arrhythmic death [13].

Thus, patients with ventricular tachyarrhythmias (VT or VF), not secondary to a transient or reversible cause, meet a Class I indication for ICD therapy. In addition, patients with syncope and significant documented VT/VF also meet indications for ICD therapy (Level of Evidence A) [14].

However it is worth noting that, in most centers, the deployment of an ICD for primary prevention far exceeds the number of devices placed for secondary prevention.

Compared to optimal medical therapy, the use of ICDs in recent trials for primary prophylaxis in CHD population was associated with a reduction in 5-year all-cause mortality of 23% to 36% and a reduction in absolute mortality of 1.5% to 3% per year.

2. Clinical parameters

Coronary disease is the main etiology of heart disease in Western countries and the major cause of heart failure and SCD.It is defined by the presence of significant coronary stenosis in a main coronary vessel or by the demonstration of previous MI.

Sudden death associated with CHD may occur in the acute context or months to years after MI. At least 50% of all SCDs due to CHD occur as a first clinical event and among subgroups of patients thought to be at relatively low risk for SCD [15].

SCD risk is associated with the conventional risk factors for coronary atherosclerosis [16] including obesity, smoking [17], genetic predisposition [18], [19], ECG pattern of LVH or LBBB, certain angiographic parameters or heart rate profile during exercise [20].

The rhythm most often recorded at the time of sudden cardiac arrest is VT or VF [21]. The pathophysiological mechanism underlying the arrhythmias can be variable and multifactorial.

Transient factors may interact with a fixed substrate that, in ischemic heart disease, is attributed to scar-based re-entry.

In chronic stage of CHD, the occurrence of SCD has an inverse relation with EF of left ventricle and, at present, this is the parameter most widely used to categorize "high risk" patients for SCD.

Other factors that have been demonstrated to contribute to the risk for SCD after MI include the presence of non-sustained ventricular tachycardia (nsVT), inducible VT by EP testing

[22] or symptomatic heart failure (HF). Premature ventricular complexes (PVC) predict an increased risk of SCD during long-term follow-up, especially if ≥ 10 PVC per hour. The presence of frequent PVCs during or after exercise has been associated with greater risk for serious cardiovascular events but not specifically SCD.

Several other parameters are considered predictors of sudden death, but all with low or moderate predictive values, whose sensitivity and specificity have not yet been studied in detail in large patient populations.

Different noninvasive exams that allow quantification of ischemia (cardiac SPECT) [23], characterization of longitudinal strain abnormalities (echocardiography) [24] or MI scar (Cardiac Magnetic Resonance) [25], T wave alternant (ECG) or the presence and extent of sympathetic denervation(cardiac ^{123}I-MIBG imaging) were used in order to improve risk stratification of sudden death in ischemic cardiomyopathy [26], [27].

3. Primary prevention trials

To date, seven multicenter studies were essential for defining the criteria and timing for ICD implantation in ischemic heart disease: Multicenter Automatic Defibrillator Implantation Trial (MADIT [28]), Coronary Artery Bypass Graft Patch (CABG-Patch) [29], Multicenter Unsustained Tachycardia Trial (MUSTT) [30], MADIT II [31], Defibrillators In Acute Myocardial Infarction Trial (DINAMIT) [32], Sudden Cardiac Death in Heart Failure (SCD-HeFT)[8] and Immediate Risk Stratification Improves Survival (IRIS) [33].

Low LV ejection fraction (up to 30 to 40%) was the inclusion criterion similar in all of these studies.

Specific criteria in each of the studies were the presence of non sustained ventricular tachycardia and electrophysiological study showing inducible VT (MADIT and MUSTT), recent coronary revascularization and abnormal signal-averaged ECG (CABG-Patch), recent MI (DINAMIT, IRIS) and heart failure (SCD-HeFT).

Based on these trials, the American College of Cardiology, American Heart Association and the European Society of Cardiology guidelines recommend the implementation of ICDs in all patients with an ejection fraction inferior or equal to 30%, as well as patients with EF less than 35% with heart failure New York Heart Association (NYHA) class II or III. ICD can be considered in postinfarction patients with EF to 40% who have sustained ventricular arrhythmias inducible during electrophysiology study [14].

As a rule, ICD implantation is not indicated in patients recovering from an acute MI (less than 40 days) or CABG surgery (within 90 days) or in patients with NYHA class IV.

The Number needed to treat (NNT) of ICD implantation in quite different between the trials depending on the severity of the patients evaluated and varied between 4 in MUSTT and 14 in SCD-HeFT [34].

There is still a controversy regarding the effect of Cardiac Resynchronization Therapy (CRT) on the risk of ventricular tachyarrhythmias, specially in patients at higher risk of heart failure [36].Some studies suggested that epicardial activation in CRT may cause dispersion of depolarization and prolongation of QT interval [37].

Recently, MADIT-CRT trial showed an inverse association between reverse remodeling and the risk of subsequent ventricular tachyarrhythmias: in high responders to resynchronization therapy (defined as ≥25% reduction in LVESD), there was a 55% lower risk of arrhythmias at 1-year post-implantation.

It seems that reverse remodeling had a dual effect of both heart failure and arrhythmia risk reduction [38].

4. ECG measurements

Classically, the presence of Left Bundle Branch Block (LBBB) was considered of major prognostic importance, associated with the occurrence of sudden death in patients with ischemic heart disease. This was based on earlier studies, most of them performed before the era of percutaneous coronary revascularization [39].

In more recent investigations, especially those resulting from secondary analyses of MUSTT and MADIT-II trials, it has become clear that QRS prolongation is related with mortality after MI, although the magnitude of the relationship between abnormal intraventricular conduction and SCD in CHD remains unclear [40].

In an analysis of MUSTT trial, the authors noted that patients with LBBB had lower ejection fractions and higher incidence of symptomatic heart failure, suggesting that the increase in overall mortality was probably due to a sicker population [41].

In the MADIT-II cohort with prolonged QRS its duration (QRSd) was found to be an independent predictor of SCD in medically managed patients (HR 2.12) but not in ICD-treated patients (HR 0.77).This was attributed to the fact that ICD-treated MADIT II patients died predominantly of non-sudden HF, and QRSd would not predict HF mortality [42]

In the cardiac resynchronization therapy trial (MADIT-CRT), CRT dramatically reduces the progression of HF in patients with a low ejection fraction and a wide QRS complex. QRS duration and morphology was considered an important prognostic factor indicating more advanced cardiac pathology [43].

Other electrocardiographic parameters in which the prognostic value was evaluated were T-wave alternant (MTWA), the signal-averaged ECG (SAECG) and QT parameters and dynamics [44].

One of the parameters with more consistent results was MTWA. TWA consist of a fluctuation of the amplitude or morphology of the T wave every other beat assessed during exercise testing or atria pacing [45].

A positive MTWA determined an approximately 2.5-fold higher risk of cardiac death and life-threatening arrhythmia and showed a very high negative predictive value both in ischemic [46] and no ischemic patients . According to guidelines, it is a recommendation class IIa the use of TWA to improve the diagnosis and risk stratification of patients with ventricular arrhythmias [14].

In a small study in patients post-MI and EF less than or equal to 30%, microvolt TWA was better than QRS duration at identifying a high-risk group and also a low-risk group unlikely to benefit from ICD therapy [47].

SAECG permits the identification of low-amplitude signals (microvolt level) at the end of the QRS complex referred to as late potentials. These indicate regions of abnormal myocardium with slow conduction believed to serve as markers of the substrate for reentrant ventricular tachyarrhythmias [48]. It has a high negative predictive value but its value is lower after coronary revascularization. [49]

5. Autonomic variables

The main variables studied included the autonomic heart rate variability (HRV)/turbulence and the baroreceptor sensitivity.

HRV corresponds to a beat-to-beat variance in cardiac cycle length resulting from the sympatho-vagal influence on the sinus node. HRV is a term that encompasses a large number of different measures derived from 24-h Holter recordings.

In general, if such measures are extremely low, it is considered that there is autonomic dysfunction and this has been shown to independently predict the risk of SCD in post-infarct patients [50].

Methods based on non linear dynamics and HR turbulence seams to provide better prognostic information than the traditional ones [51], [52].

Several studies have evaluated the prognostic value of heart rate variability in patients with ischemic heart disease [53]. In the randomized defibrillator in AMI trial (DYNAMIT), which used reduced SDNN combined with reduced left ventricular ejection fraction measured early (within 2weeks) after AMI as an inclusion criterion, there was no mortality benefit from ICD therapy in these presumably high risk patients [32].

On the contrary, in the cardiac arrhythmias and risk stratification after myocardial infarction (CARISMA) study, reduced HR variability measured at 6weeks after AMI, particularly the very-low frequency spectral component, was a powerful index in predicting arrhythmic events. The REFINE trial (Risk estimation after infarction, non-invasive evaluation) confirmed that HRV and HR turbulence yield more powerful prognostic information for arrhythmic events when measured later (6–10weeks) after AMI [54].

Despite these promising results, further prospective studies are needed to determine the usefulness of these parameters in clinical practice.

Reduced baroreflex sensivity, a quantitative index of primarily vagal reflexes, evaluated by the phenylephrine method or by a non-invasive measurement [55], is also useful in assessing the risk of SCD [56, 57].

6. Autonomic imaging

There is evidence that regional and global sympathetic denervation could predispose to ventricular arrhythmias in post-MI patients. The denervated but viable myocardium could be hyperresponsive to circulating catecholamines [58, 59].

Using imaging methods for the evaluation of the sympathetic system in vivo, in human and animal models, such as [12^{13}I-mIBG cardiac imaging, it has been reported that the mismatch between sympathetic innervation and perfusion could be associated with increased risk of ventricular arrhythmias.

The extent of sympathetic denervation measured at 4-Hour delayed ^{123}I-mIBG SPECT imaging has been correlated with inducibility of ventricular arrhythmias in electrophysiological testing [60]. In another study including patients with advanced heart failure, late [12^{13}I-MIBG SPECT defect score was also an independent predictor for ventricular arrhythmias causing appropriate ICD therapy (primary end point) as well as the composite of appropriate ICD therapy or cardiac death (secondary end point) [27]

More studies are required to determine the role of autonomic imaging in post-MI patients, possibly detailing their correlation with CMR findings.

7. Electrophysiological testing

Patients after MI have the highest induction rates in electrophysiological study and the presence of ejection fraction less than 40% and asymptomatic NSVT is associated with a inducibility of 20-40% [22], [61].

Programmed ventricular stimulation identifies most patients at risk for sustained monomorphic ventricular tachycardia associated with reentrant circuits that result of the healing process after infarction [22].

Electrophysiological study was required in MADIT, MUSTT, BEST–ICD [62], but not in MADIT –II and SCD-HeFt trials.

Based on these trials, electrophysiological testing is not required before ICD implantation. It is recommended (class I) for diagnostic evaluation of symptoms suggestive of tachyarrhythmias, to guide VT ablation and for differential diagnosis of a wide-QRS-complex tachycardias of unclear mechanism [14].

Electrophysiological study is also reasonable for risk stratification in patients with NSVT, and LVEF equal or less than 40% (Class IIa). Inducibility of VT in patients with NSVT is associated with a high risk for VT/FV and the characteristics of NSVT could not predict the inducibility [63].

8. Echocardiographic parameters

The echocardiogram is a fundamental exam for the identification of candidates for ICD implantation. Although an LVEF of <40% is commonly used for stratification of patients at risk for ventricular arrhythmias, it does not allow accurate discrimination of patients with or without sudden arrhythmic death. Moreover, sudden arrhythmic death also occurs in patients with an LVEF of ≥40% [64].

The technical advances in echocardiography will probably allow exploring the appraisal value of new variables beyond the ejection fraction of the left ventricle in the risk stratification.

In a unicenter study a greater involvement of peri-infarct zone longitudinal strain was independently associated with an increased risk of having an appropriate ICD therapy on follow-up. In such study the odds of dying in a patient with a peri-infarct zone strain value of -6% was approximately 11.5 times that of a patient with a peri-infarct zone strain value of -17% [65].

9. Cardiac magnetic resonance

Cardiac MRI allows characterization of cardiac morphology in patients with poor echo cardiographic window and provides an estimate of the location and amount of intramyocardial fibrosis.

The presence of myocardial scar or fibrosis as measured by delayed enhancement after administration of gadolinium has been recently associated with post-infarct arrhythmic death [66], [67] suggesting that contrast-enhanced MRI may enable better risk stratification for ICD implantation among patients with prior MI compared with traditional variables such as LVEF and NYHA class.

Roes S et al identified infarct tissue heterogeneity on contrast-enhanced MRI as a strong predictor of spontaneous ventricular arrhythmia in ICD therapy recipients [68]. In a more recent study from a tertiary center which included the monitoring of 52 patients, it was identified a relationship between the transmurality of infarction and the occurrence of spontaneous ventricular arrhythmias in patients with chronic ischemic cardiopathy [69].

10. Conclusion

Ischemic heart disease is the heart disease in which most often there is indication for an ICD implantation. However, after placed, these devices are used in a minority of patients in the context of primary prevention.

Left ventricular dysfunction remains the most robust parameter in the decision to implant an ICD. All therapeutic measures that can accelerate or improve myocardial reperfusion by contributing to the preservation of ventricular function are undoubtedly the best strategies to reduce costs associated with ICDs.

In recent years numerous studies have been performed using non-invasive methods for diagnosis of autonomic dysfunction or anatomic-functional abnormalities but it remains a need for a proper validation of predictors of arrhythmic death.

Author details

Elisabete Martins

Address all correspondence to: ebernardes@med.up.pt

Department of Medicine; Porto Medical School, Portugal

References

[1] Buxton AE, Calkins H, Callans DJ, DiMarco JP, Fisher JD, Greene HL, et al. ACC/AHA/HRS 2006 key data elements and definitions for electrophysiological studies and procedures: a report of the American College of Cardiology/American Heart Association Task Force on Clinical Data Standards (ACC/AHA/HRS Writing Committee to Develop Data Standards on Electrophysiology). Circulation. 2006; 114(23): 2534-70.

[2] Jimenez RA, Myerburg RJ. Sudden cardiac death. Magnitude of the problem, substrate/trigger interaction, and populations at high risk. Cardiol Clin. 1993; 11(1): 1-9.

[3] Priori SG, Aliot E, Blomstrom-Lundqvist C, Bossaert L, Breithardt G, Brugada P, et al. Update of the guidelines on sudden cardiac death of the European Society of Cardiology. Eur Heart J. 2003; 24(1): 13-5.

[4] Barbour DJ, Warnes CA, Roberts WC. Cardiac findings associated with sudden death secondary to atherosclerotic coronary artery disease: comparison of patients with and those without previous angina pectoris and/or healed myocardial infarction. Circulation. 1987; 75(3 Pt 2): II9-11.

[5] Goldberger JJ, Cain ME, Hohnloser SH, Kadish AH, Knight BP, Lauer MS, et al. American Heart Association/American College of Cardiology Foundation/Heart Rhythm Society scientific statement on noninvasive risk stratification techniques for identifying patients at risk for sudden cardiac death: a scientific statement from the American Heart Association Council on Clinical Cardiology Committee on Electro-

cardiography and Arrhythmias and Council on Epidemiology and Prevention. Circulation. 2008; 118(14): 1497-518.

[6] Hjalmarson A. Effects of beta blockade on sudden cardiac death during acute myocardial infarction and the postinfarction period. Am J Cardiol. 1997; 80(9B): 35J-9J.

[7] Waldo AL, Camm AJ, deRuyter H, Friedman PL, MacNeil DJ, Pauls JF, et al. Effect of d-sotalol on mortality in patients with left ventricular dysfunction after recent and remote myocardial infarction. The SWORD Investigators. Survival With Oral d-Sotalol. Lancet. 1996; 348(9019): 7-12.

[8] Mark DB, Nelson CL, Anstrom KJ, Al-Khatib SM, Tsiatis AA, Cowper PA, et al. Cost-effectiveness of defibrillator therapy or amiodarone in chronic stable heart failure: results from the Sudden Cardiac Death in Heart Failure Trial (SCD-HeFT). Circulation. 2006; 114(2): 135-42.

[9] Weaver WD, Cobb LA, Hallstrom AP, Fahrenbruch C, Copass MK, Ray R. Factors influencing survival after out-of-hospital cardiac arrest. J Am Coll Cardiol. 1986; 7(4): 752-7.

[10] A comparison of antiarrhythmic-drug therapy with implantable defibrillators in patients resuscitated from near-fatal ventricular arrhythmias. The Antiarrhythmics versus Implantable Defibrillators (AVID) Investigators. N Engl J Med. 1997; 337(22): 1576-83.

[11] Connolly SJ, Gent M, Roberts RS, Dorian P, Roy D, Sheldon RS, et al. Canadian implantable defibrillator study (CIDS) : a randomized trial of the implantable cardioverter defibrillator against amiodarone. Circulation. 2000; 101(11): 1297-302.

[12] Kuck KH, Cappato R, Siebels J, Ruppel R. Randomized comparison of antiarrhythmic drug therapy with implantable defibrillators in patients resuscitated from cardiac arrest : the Cardiac Arrest Study Hamburg (CASH). Circulation. 2000; 102(7): 748-54.

[13] Connolly SJ, Hallstrom AP, Cappato R, Schron EB, Kuck KH, Zipes DP, et al. Meta-analysis of the implantable cardioverter defibrillator secondary prevention trials. AVID, CASH and CIDS studies. Antiarrhythmics vs Implantable Defibrillator study. Cardiac Arrest Study Hamburg . Canadian Implantable Defibrillator Study. Eur Heart J. 2000; 21(24): 2071-8.

[14] Zipes DP, Camm AJ, Borggrefe M, Buxton AE, Chaitman B, Fromer M, et al. ACC/AHA/ESC 2006 guidelines for management of patients with ventricular arrhythmias and the prevention of sudden cardiac death: a report of the American College of Cardiology/American Heart Association Task Force and the European Society of Cardiology Committee for Practice Guidelines (Writing Committee to Develop Guidelines for Management of Patients With Ventricular Arrhythmias and the Prevention of Sudden Cardiac Death). J Am Coll Cardiol. 2006; 48(5): e247-346.

[15] Myerburg RJ. Sudden cardiac death: exploring the limits of our knowledge. J Cardiovasc Electrophysiol. 2001; 12(3): 369-81.

[16] Holmes DR, Jr., Davis K, Gersh BJ, Mock MB, Pettinger MB. Risk factor profiles of patients with sudden cardiac death and death from other cardiac causes: a report from the Coronary Artery Surgery Study (CASS). J Am Coll Cardiol. 1989; 13(3): 524-30.

[17] Kannel WB, Thomas HE, Jr. Sudden coronary death: the Framingham Study. Ann N Y Acad Sci. 1982; 382: 3-21.

[18] Snapir A, Mikkelsson J, Perola M, Penttila A, Scheinin M, Karhunen PJ. Variation in the alpha2B-adrenoceptor gene as a risk factor for prehospital fatal myocardial infarction and sudden cardiac death. J Am Coll Cardiol. 2003; 41(2): 190-4.

[19] Friedlander Y, Siscovick DS, Weinmann S, Austin MA, Psaty BM, Lemaitre RN, et al. Family history as a risk factor for primary cardiac arrest. Circulation. 1998; 97(2): 155-60.

[20] Jouven X, Empana JP, Schwartz PJ, Desnos M, Courbon D, Ducimetiere P. Heart-rate profile during exercise as a predictor of sudden death. N Engl J Med. 2005; 352(19): 1951-8.

[21] Luu M, Stevenson WG, Stevenson LW, Baron K, Walden J. Diverse mechanisms of unexpected cardiac arrest in advanced heart failure. Circulation. 1989; 80(6): 1675-80.

[22] Buxton AE, Lee KL, DiCarlo L, Gold MR, Greer GS, Prystowsky EN, et al. Electrophysiologic testing to identify patients with coronary artery disease who are at risk for sudden death. Multicenter Unsustained Tachycardia Trial Investigators. N Engl J Med. 2000; 342(26): 1937-45.

[23] Piccini JP, Horton JR, Shaw LK, Al-Khatib SM, Lee KL, Iskandrian AE, et al. Single-photon emission computed tomography myocardial perfusion defects are associated with an increased risk of all-cause death, cardiovascular death, and sudden cardiac death. Circ Cardiovasc Imaging. 2008; 1(3): 180-8.

[24] Yan GH, Wang M, Yiu KH, Lau CP, Zhi G, Lee SW, et al. Subclinical left ventricular dysfunction revealed by circumferential 2D strain imaging in patients with coronary artery disease and fragmented QRS complex. Heart Rhythm. 2012; 9(6): 928-35.

[25] Scott PA, Morgan JM, Carroll N, Murday DC, Roberts PR, Peebles CR, et al. The extent of left ventricular scar quantified by late gadolinium enhancement MRI is associated with spontaneous ventricular arrhythmias in patients with coronary artery disease and implantable cardioverter-defibrillators. Circ Arrhythm Electrophysiol. 2011; 4(3): 324-30.

[26] Nishisato K, Hashimoto A, Nakata T, Doi T, Yamamoto H, Nagahara D, et al. Impaired cardiac sympathetic innervation and myocardial perfusion are related to lethal arrhythmia: quantification of cardiac tracers in patients with ICDs. J Nucl Med. 2010; 51(8): 1241-9.

[27] Boogers MJ, Borleffs CJ, Henneman MM, van Bommel RJ, van Ramshorst J, Boersma E, et al. Cardiac sympathetic denervation assessed with 123-iodine metaiodobenzylguanidine imaging predicts ventricular arrhythmias in implantable cardioverter-defibrillator patients. J Am Coll Cardiol. 2010; 55(24): 2769-77.

[28] Moss AJ, Hall WJ, Cannom DS, Daubert JP, Higgins SL, Klein H, et al. Improved survival with an implanted defibrillator in patients with coronary disease at high risk for ventricular arrhythmia. Multicenter Automatic Defibrillator Implantation Trial Investigators. N Engl J Med. 1996; 335(26): 1933-40.

[29] Bigger JT, Jr. Prophylactic use of implanted cardiac defibrillators in patients at high risk for ventricular arrhythmias after coronary-artery bypass graft surgery. Coronary Artery Bypass Graft (CABG) Patch Trial Investigators. N Engl J Med. 1997; 337(22): 1569-75.

[30] Lee KL, Hafley G, Fisher JD, Gold MR, Prystowsky EN, Talajic M, et al. Effect of implantable defibrillators on arrhythmic events and mortality in the multicenter unsustained tachycardia trial. Circulation. 2002; 106(2): 233-8.

[31] Moss AJ, Zareba W, Hall WJ, Klein H, Wilber DJ, Cannom DS, et al. Prophylactic implantation of a defibrillator in patients with myocardial infarction and reduced ejection fraction. N Engl J Med. 2002; 346(12): 877-83.

[32] Hohnloser SH, Kuck KH, Dorian P, Roberts RS, Hampton JR, Hatala R, et al. Prophylactic use of an implantable cardioverter-defibrillator after acute myocardial infarction. N Engl J Med. 2004; 351(24): 2481-8.

[33] Steinbeck G, Andresen D, Seidl K, Brachmann J, Hoffmann E, Wojciechowski D, et al. Defibrillator implantation early after myocardial infarction. N Engl J Med. 2009; 361(15): 1427-36.

[34] Mountantonakis SE, Hutchinson MD. Indications for implantable cardioverter-defibrillator placement in ischemic cardiomyopathy and after myocardial infarction. Curr Heart Fail Rep. 2011; 8(4): 252-9.

[35] Goldenberg I, Gillespie J, Moss AJ, Hall WJ, Klein H, McNitt S, et al. Long-term benefit of primary prevention with an implantable cardioverter-defibrillator: an extended 8-year follow-up study of the Multicenter Automatic Defibrillator Implantation Trial II. Circulation. 2010; 122(13): 1265-71.

[36] Barsheshet A, Moss AJ, Huang DT, McNitt S, Zareba W, Goldenberg I. Applicability of a risk score for prediction of the long-term (8-year) benefit of the implantable cardioverter-defibrillator. J Am Coll Cardiol. 2012; 59(23): 2075-9.

[37] Medina-Ravell VA, Lankipalli RS, Yan GX, Antzelevitch C, Medina-Malpica NA, Medina-Malpica OA, et al. Effect of epicardial or biventricular pacing to prolong QT interval and increase transmural dispersion of repolarization: does resynchronization therapy pose a risk for patients predisposed to long QT or torsade de pointes? Circulation. 2003; 107(5): 740-6.

[38] Barsheshet A, Wang PJ, Moss AJ, Solomon SD, Al-Ahmad A, McNitt S, et al. Reverse remodeling and the risk of ventricular tachyarrhythmias in the MADIT-CRT (Multicenter Automatic Defibrillator Implantation Trial-Cardiac Resynchronization Therapy). J Am Coll Cardiol. 2011; 57(24): 2416-23.

[39] Brilakis ES, Wright RS, Kopecky SL, Reeder GS, Williams BA, Miller WL. Bundle branch block as a predictor of long-term survival after acute myocardial infarction. Am J Cardiol, 2001; 88:205–209.

[40] Brenyo A, Zareba W. Prognostic significance of QRS duration and morphology. Cardiol J. 2011; 18(1): 8-17.

[41] Zimetbaum PJ, Buxton AE, Batsford W, Fisher JD, Hafley GE, Lee KL, et al. Electrocardiographic predictors of arrhythmic death and total mortality in the multicenter unsustained tachycardia trial. Circulation. 2004; 110(7): 766-9.

[42] Dhar R, Alsheikh-Ali AA, Estes NA, 3rd, Moss AJ, Zareba W, Daubert JP, et al. Association of prolonged QRS duration with ventricular tachyarrhythmias and sudden cardiac death in the Multicenter Automatic Defibrillator Implantation Trial II (MADIT-II). Heart Rhythm. 2008; 5(6): 807-13.

[43] Goldenberg I, Moss AJ, Hall WJ, Foster E, Goldberger JJ, Santucci P, et al. Predictors of response to cardiac resynchronization therapy in the Multicenter Automatic Defibrillator Implantation Trial with Cardiac Resynchronization Therapy (MADIT-CRT). Circulation. 2011; 124(14): 1527-36.

[44] Jensen BT, Abildstrom SZ, Larroude CE, Agner E, Torp-Pedersen C, Nyvad O, et al. QT dynamics in risk stratification after myocardial infarction. Heart Rhythm. 2005; 2(4): 357-64.

[45] Ikeda T, Saito H, Tanno K, Shimizu H, Watanabe J, Ohnishi Y, et al. T-wave alternans as a predictor for sudden cardiac death after myocardial infarction. Am J Cardiol. 2002; 89(1): 79-82.

[46] Chow T, Kereiakes DJ, Bartone C, Booth T, Schloss EJ, Waller T, et al. Prognostic utility of microvolt T-wave alternans in risk stratification of patients with ischemic cardiomyopathy. J Am Coll Cardiol. 2006; 47(9): 1820-7.

[47] Bloomfield DM, Steinman RC, Namerow PB, Parides M, Davidenko J, Kaufman ES, et al. Microvolt T-wave alternans distinguishes between patients likely and patients not likely to benefit from implanted cardiac defibrillator therapy: a solution to the Multicenter Automatic Defibrillator Implantation Trial (MADIT) II conundrum. Circulation. 2004; 110(14): 1885-9.

[48] Steinberg JS, Prystowsky E, Freedman RA, Moreno F, Katz R, Kron J, et al. Use of the signal-averaged electrocardiogram for predicting inducible ventricular tachycardia in patients with unexplained syncope: relation to clinical variables in a multivariate analysis. J Am Coll Cardiol. 1994; 23(1): 99-106.

[49] Cook JR, Flack JE, Gregory CA, Deaton DW, Rousou JA, Engelman RM. Influence of the preoperative signal-averaged electrocardiogram on left ventricular function after coronary artery bypass graft surgery in patients with left ventricular dysfunction. The CABG Patch Trial. Am J Cardiol. 1998; 82(3): 285-9.

[50] Zuanetti G, Neilson JM, Latini R, Santoro E, Maggioni AP, Ewing DJ. Prognostic significance of heart rate variability in post-myocardial infarction patients in the fibrinolytic era. The GISSI-2 results. Gruppo Italiano per lo Studio della Sopravvivenza nell' Infarto Miocardico. Circulation. 1996; 94(3): 432-6.

[51] Bauer A, Malik M, Schmidt G, Barthel P, Bonnemeier H, Cygankiewicz I, et al. Heart rate turbulence: standards of measurement, physiological interpretation, and clinical use: International Society for Holter and Noninvasive Electrophysiology Consensus. J Am Coll Cardiol. 2008; 52(17): 1353-65.

[52] Perkiomaki JS, Jokinen V, Tapanainen J, Airaksinen KE, Huikuri HV. Autonomic markers as predictors of nonfatal acute coronary events after myocardial infarction. Ann Noninvasive Electrocardiol. 2008; 13(2): 120-9.

[53] Huikuri HV, Stein PK. Clinical application of heart rate variability after acute myocardial infarction. Front Physiol. 2012; 3: 41.

[54] Huikuri HV, Exner DV, Kavanagh KM, Aggarwal SG, Mitchell LB, Messier MD, et al. Attenuated recovery of heart rate turbulence early after myocardial infarction identifies patients at high risk for fatal or near-fatal arrhythmic events. Heart Rhythm. 2010; 7(2): 229-35.

[55] Pinna GD, La Rovere MT, Maestri R, Mortara A, Bigger JT, Schwartz PJ. Comparison between invasive and non-invasive measurements of baroreflex sensitivity; implications for studies on risk stratification after a myocardial infarction. Eur Heart J. 2000; 21(18): 1522-9.

[56] La Rovere MT, Pinna GD, Hohnloser SH, Marcus FI, Mortara A, Nohara R, et al. Baroreflex sensitivity and heart rate variability in the identification of patients at risk for life-threatening arrhythmias: implications for clinical trials. Circulation. 2001; 103(16): 2072-7.

[57] Farrell TG, Odemuyiwa O, Bashir Y, Cripps TR, Malik M, Ward DE, et al. Prognostic value of baroreflex sensitivity testing after acute myocardial infarction. Br Heart J. 1992; 67(2): 129-37.

[58] Podrid PJ, Fuchs T, Candinas R. Role of the sympathetic nervous system in the genesis of ventricular arrhythmia. Circulation. 1990; 82(2 Suppl): I103-13.

[59] Kammerling JJ, Green FJ, Watanabe AM, Inoue H, Barber MJ, Henry DP, et al. Denervation supersensitivity of refractoriness in noninfarcted areas apical to transmural myocardial infarction. Circulation. 1987; 76(2): 383-93.

[60] Bax JJ, Kraft O, Buxton AE, Fjeld JG, Parizek P, Agostini D, et al. 123 I-mIBG scintigraphy to predict inducibility of ventricular arrhythmias on cardiac electrophysiology

testing: a prospective multicenter pilot study. Circ Cardiovasc Imaging. 2008; 1(2): 131-40.

[61] Swerdlow CD, Bardy GH, McAnulty J, Kron J, Lee JT, Graham E, et al. Determinants of induced sustained arrhythmias in survivors of out-of-hospital ventricular fibrillation. Circulation. 1987; 76(5): 1053-60.

[62] Raviele A, Bongiorni MG, Brignole M, Cappato R, Capucci A, Gaita F, et al. Early EPS/ICD strategy in survivors of acute myocardial infarction with severe left ventricular dysfunction on optimal beta-blocker treatment. The BEta-blocker STrategy plus ICD trial. Europace. 2005; 7(4): 327-37.

[63] Buxton AE, Lee KL, DiCarlo L, Echt DS, Fisher JD, Greer GS, et al. Nonsustained ventricular tachycardia in coronary artery disease: relation to inducible sustained ventricular tachycardia. MUSTT Investigators. Ann Intern Med. 1996; 125(1): 35-9.

[64] Goldberger JJ, Cain ME, Hohnloser SH, Kadish AH, Knight BP, Lauer MS, et al. American Heart Association/American College of Cardiology Foundation/Heart Rhythm Society Scientific Statement on Noninvasive Risk Stratification Techniques for Identifying Patients at Risk for Sudden Cardiac Death. A scientific statement from the American Heart Association Council on Clinical Cardiology Committee on Electrocardiography and Arrhythmias and Council on Epidemiology and Prevention. J Am Coll Cardiol. 2008; 52(14): 1179-99.

[65] Ng AC, Bertini M, Borleffs CJ, Delgado V, Boersma E, Piers SR, et al. Predictors of death and occurrence of appropriate implantable defibrillator therapies in patients with ischemic cardiomyopathy. Am J Cardiol. 2010; 106(11): 1566-73.

[66] Klem I, Weinsaft JW, Bahnson TD, Hegland D, Kim HW, Hayes B, et al. Assessment of myocardial scarring improves risk stratification in patients evaluated for cardiac defibrillator implantation. J Am Coll Cardiol. 2012; 60(5): 408-20.

[67] Gao P, Yee R, Gula L, Krahn AD, Skanes A, Leong-Sit P, et al. Prediction of arrhythmic events in ischemic and dilated cardiomyopathy patients referred for implantable cardiac defibrillator: evaluation of multiple scar quantification measures for late gadolinium enhancement magnetic resonance imaging. Circ Cardiovasc Imaging. 2012; 5(4): 448-56.

[68] Roes SD, Borleffs CJ, van der Geest RJ, Westenberg JJ, Marsan NA, Kaandorp TA, et al. Infarct tissue heterogeneity assessed with contrast-enhanced MRI predicts spontaneous ventricular arrhythmia in patients with ischemic cardiomyopathy and implantable cardioverter-defibrillator. Circ Cardiovasc Imaging. 2009; 2(3): 183-90.

[69] Boye P, Abdel-Aty H, Zacharzowsky U, Bohl S, Schwenke C, van der Geest RJ, et al. Prediction of life-threatening arrhythmic events in patients with chronic myocardial infarction by contrast-enhanced CMR. JACC Cardiovasc Imaging. 2011; 4(8): 871-9.

Chapter 4

Implantable Cardioverter-Defibrillators in Sudden Cardiac Death Prevention: What Guidelines Don't Tell

Marzia Giaccardi, Andrea Colella,
Giovanni Maria Santoro, Alfredo Zuppiroli and
Gian Franco Gensini

Additional information is available at the end of the chapter

http://dx.doi.org/10.5772/52840

1. Introduction

A *guideline* is a statement by which to determine a course of action. A guideline aims to streamline particular processes according to a set routine or sound practice. By definition, following a guideline is never mandatory. Guidelines are not binding and are not enforced [5]. In effect guidelines are derived from 3 sources of data: 1. randomized clinical trials; 2. observational data from cohorts of high-risk patients with less common diseases; and 3. expert opinion on potential benefit for clinical condition or specific circumstances in which data are limited or uncertain. For all 3 categories of clinical guidance, there are limitations in available data that reinforce the importance of physician judgment in decision making, based on circumstances of individual cases or subgroups of patients [6]. Understanding the value and limitations of current information is important not only for the clinical electrophysiologist, but also for general cardiologists and primary care physicians because of their roles in referring appropriate patients for consideration of implantable cardioverter- defibrillator therapy and for the clinical management of patients at risk of sudden cardiac death. While the high stakes and unpredictable nature of sudden cardiac death justifiably provoke fear and uncertainty, emotional factors should not outweigh scientific evidence. In this context the obligation to adhere to guidelines could, in effects, to have paradoxically dulled our discriminatory senses as clinicians [7].

2. Sudden cardiac death

Sudden cardiac death (SCD) is generally defined as a sudden and unexpected death from a cardiovascular cause in a person with or without preexisting heart disease. The specificity of this definition varies depending on whether the event was witnessed; however, most studies include cases that are associated with a witnessed collapse, death occurring within 1 hour of an acute change in clinical status, or an unexpected death that occurred within the previous 24 hours [8-10]. Despite the significant decline in coronary artery disease (CAD), the overall burden of SCD in the population remains high. In the second half of the 20th century, SCD continues to claim 250.000 to 300.000 US lives annualy [11,12]. In North America and Europe the annual incidence of SCD ranges between 50 to 100 per 100.000 in the general population [13-16]. However, even in the presence of advanced first responder systems for resuscitation of out-of-hospital cardiac arrest, the overall survival to hospital discharge was recently estimated to be only 7,9% [17]. In addition, the majority of SCDs occur at home, often where the event is unwitnessed [18,19]. SCD can manifest as ventricular tachycardia (VT), ventricular fibrillation (VF), that accounting for approximately three-quarters of cases, the rest 25% caused by bradyarrhythmias or asystole [20-22]. In a significant proportion of patients, SCD can present without warning or a recognized triggering mechanism. The mean age of those affected is in the mid 60s, and at least 40% of patients will suffer SCD before the age of 65 [14].There is also strong evidence from studies in North America and Europe that there are significantly altered trends in the presenting arrhythmia observed by first responders among SCD cases [23,24]. The prevalence of SCD cases presenting with VF is decreasing with a corresponding increase in the proportion of cases presenting with pulseless electric activity (PEA). Given the extremes of resuscitation outcome based on presenting arrhythmia (>25% survival for VF and <2% for PEA) [14], it is important to improve our understanding of the determinants of these altered trends. Moreover for some segments of the population rate of SCD are not decreasing and may actually be increasing [23, 25].

More recent studies suggest that the incidence of VF or VT as the first recorded rhythm in out-of-hospital cardiac arrest has declined to perhaps even <30% in the past several decades [17,23,26]. The risk of SCD in myocardial infarction (MI) survivors has also declined significantly over the past 30 years, presumably due to early reperfusion and optimal medical therapy practices [27]. Recurrent ischemia may not be significantly associated with SCD, whereas heart failure due to MI markedly increases the risk of SCD [27]. Interestingly, acute ischemia is an established cause of VF and polymorphic VT [28], whereas cardiac death in patients with nonischemic dilated cardiomyopathy and functional class IV heart failure is more often due to bradyarrhythmia or electromechanical dissociation than due to ventricular tachyarrhythmias [29].

As a result, automated external defibrillators (ICD), which improve resuscitation rates for witnessed arrests only due to VT/VF [30], may have limited effectiveness on reducing overall mortality from SCD because SCD represent a current epidemic that is not exclusively due to ventricular tachyarrhythmias. These observations may have important implications when considering both secondary and primary SCD prevention by implantable ICDs [31].

http://dx.doi.org/10.5772/52840

3. Implantable cardioverter defibrillator

The ICD has emerged as a generally accepted therapy for prevention of SCD in selected categories of patients. Nearly 4 decades elapsed between the original notion that an ICD might be a useful clinical strategy, its subsequent development, and its current acceptance in various clinical settings based on randomized trial data. Each decade played a distinctive role in the evolution of ICD therapy. From the late 1960s until the first patient implant in 1980 [32], Mirowski's concept of a "standby automatic defibrillator" [33,34] met with skepticism [35] and concern about the practical difficulties in designing and manufacturing such a device [36,37]. After the first human device implant in 1980, clinical acceptance of the concept was initially slow, but began to accelerate after Food and Drug Administration approval in 1985 and Medicare coverage for limited indications in 1986. The early scientific support for the clinical value of the ICD was limited to a series of nonrandomized observational studies involving cohorts of high-risk patients. They were counterbalanced by contemporary interest in studies exploring the value of antiarrhythmic drug therapy guided by ambulatory arrhythmia monitoring or electrophysiological testing, and antiarrhythmic surgical techniques. This created uncertainty and intense debate in the electrophysiology community that continued even after the publication of the CAST (Cardiac Arrhythmia Suppression Trial) study [38,39] highlighted the potential dangers of empiric treatment with membrane-active antiarrhythmic drugs. Nonetheless, the CAST study was seminal in both constituting a turning point of the concept of antiarrhythmic drug therapy for prevention of SCD and serving as a catalyst for the recognition of the importance of randomized trial data to validate the potential for ICD benefit.

4. Secondary SCD prevention

The actual guidelines tell:

ICD in secondary prevention is indicated for survivors of cardiac arrest due to ventricular VF or VT and syncope and VF/VT inducible at electrophysiological study.

The first trial to investigate the use of ICD as first choice treatment in survivors of cardiac arrest compared with antiarrhythmic drugs was the Dutch study [40]. In a relatively small population of 60 patients, a strategy of ICD implantation as first-line treatment was shown to be preferable to medical therapy, conferring a significant reduction of a combined endpoint of main outcome events, included death, recurrent cardiac arrest, and cardiac transplantation. Three subsequent randomized clinical trials have evaluated the effect of ICD on overall mortality [41-43]. The AVID (Antiarrhythmics Versus Implantable Defibrillators) trial is the only trial to demonstrate statistically significant mortality reduction from ICD therapy in secondary prevention. After an interim analysis, the study was prematurely discontinued due to a 9% absolute increase in death in the antiarrhythmic group (mainly amiodarone) at 18 months (24.0% vs. 15.8%, $p=0.02$).

What the guidelines don't tell is that, although statistical adjustments were attempted, it is difficult to overlook the >3-fold utilization of beta-blockers in the ICD group (38.1% vs. 11.0% at 1 year) and the 5% higher incidence of atrial fibrillation and NYHA functional class III heart failure in the antiarrhythmic group, and lower incidence of congestive heart failure in the ICD group as additive confounding variables that amplified net clinical benefit in favor of ICD therapy. Moreover, clinical benefit was not observed in patients with an EF >35% and <20% [44]. While the number needed to treat in this trial was 11 ICD implants to save 1 life, the unadjusted improvement in mean survival was only 0.21 year, or 2.6 months (31 vs. 29 months). This small difference was reduced by 15% when adjustments were made for heart failure and EF. This modest prolongation of life was valued at $85,522 [45], which included the untoward costs of the 4% absolute increase in rehospitalizations in the ICD group (60% vs. 56%, p=0.04).

Two smaller randomized trials, the CIDS (Canadian Implantable Defibrillator Study) and CASH (Cardiac Arrest Study Hamburg) trials, failed to demonstrate statistically significant reductions in mortality with ICD therapy for secondary prevention. These findings occurred despite similar inequities of beta-blockade therapy in ICD patients in the CIDS trial, with significantly higher event rates (44.4% in the CASH trial, 29.6% in the CIDS trial, and 24.0% in the AVID trial in control arms) and longer follow-up (57 months in the CASH trial, 36 months in the CIDS trial, and 18 months in the AVID trial). By current clinical trial standards, these trials, which did not meet conventional statistical significance, may not pass muster with the Food and Drug Administration. These nonsignificant trends in favor of ICD therapy prompted a meta-analysis that showed a significant difference in mortality in favor of ICD [46]. With a combined follow-up period of 6 years, patients with defibrillators lived only 4.4 months longer than those treated with antiarrhythmic therapy, and all statistically significant differences were nonsustained, narrowing at 4 years toward negligible after 6 years. As seen in the AVID trial, patients with an EF >35% did not experience survival benefit from ICD therapy. The skeptic, therefore, might interpret these results as suggesting that ICD confers a relatively small and rather transient survival benefit for secondary prevention in patients with EF of 35-40%, and this might be lost when β-blockers is implemented [31].

5. Primary SCD prevention

The actual guidelines tell:

ICD in primary prevention is indicated for patients with EF ≤ 35% due to prior MI (at least 40 days after infarct) with NYHA class II-III heart failure (and NYHA I if EF ≤ 30%); nonischemic dilated cardiomyopathy with EF ≤ 35% and NYHA class II-III heart failure; and ischemic cardiomyopathy with EF ≤ 40% and VF/VT inducible at electrophysiological testing. These findings arise from trials which have shown that prophylactic ICD therapy may improve survival in patients with increased risk of arrhythmic death.

What the guidelines don't tell is that:

http://dx.doi.org/10.5772/52840

5.1. Limiations of studies

The Multicenter Automatic Defibrillator Implantation Trial (MADIT) and the Multicenter Unsustained Tachycardia Trial (MUSTT) have demonstrated that prophylactic ICD therapy may improve survival in patients with increased risk of arrhythmic death [47,48]. The results of this trials may not be directly applicable to current medical practice, as the overall low rate of medication administration is not in compliance with current postmyocardial infraction treatment guidelines. For instance, in the MADIT only 8% of patients in the control group and 26% of patients in the ICD group were receiving β-blockers at 1 month of follow-up. Similarly in the MUSTT only 29% of the electrophysiologically guided therapy group was on β-blockers. Moreover the highly selected MADIT population is difficult to categorize as a primary prevention group. Induction of sustained ventricular arrhythmias and procainamide suppression is rarely, if ever, performed in current practice, and this feature may have been important for identifying patients more likely to experience adverse events (mortality rate 39%). The event rate in the control arm was higher than those seen in secondary prevention trials (25,3% in AVID vs 32% in MADIT, at 2 years). The larger MADIT II study demonstrated a 5,6% absolute mortality benefit (19,8% vs 14,2%) at 20 months of follow-up in ICD arm compared with patients in conventional medical therapy [49]. This difference, the smallest difference seen in any ICD trial demonstrating statistically significant benefit, was likely attenuated by a lower risk population enrolled without spontaneous ventricular arrhythmias or induced by the electrophysiological study. In addition, the equivalent high rate of β-blockers in both arms (70%) and low rate of amiodarone therapy (13% ICD vs 10% control) were likely factors that drove the event rates lower. Several insights often overlooked in MADIT II deserve mention. When examining the subgroup analysis, patients with QRS less than 150 msec, and EF greater than 25% did not derive benefit, suggesting that a sicker subpopulation within may be most optimal for selection. These data was confirmed in a MADIT II subanalysis that showed a U-shaped curve for ICD efficacy, demonstrating that patients with the lowest and highest risk scores had attenuated benefit from ICD therapy [50]. Another item of note are an unexpected 5% absolute increase in hospitalization for new or worsened congestive heart failure seen in the ICD group (19,9% vs 14,9%). Of note, this 5% trend in increased heart failure is the exact reverse of the mortality rates and absolute overall benefit. This observation confirmed some of the initial suspicion that right ventricular pacing and ICD discharges may have deleterious effects on myocardial function [51]. Furthermore, depriving a patient of sudden death may shift the mode of death to pump failure, which has the potential to be more costly and morbid [52]. Similar phenomena were observed in the Defibrillator in Acute Myocardial Infarction Trial (DINAMIT) in which the prevention of arrhythmic death with ICD was counterbalanced by excess death from nonarrhythmic causes [53]. The potential for causal harm from ICD shocks was again suggested by a substudy that showed the increased risk from nonarrhythmic death to be confined only to those that received ICD discharges. Due to the lack of mortality benefit seen immediately after myocardial infarction, the guidelines specify a 40-day blanking period during which ICD implantation is contraindicated. The findings of DINAMIT contradict the inferences from the VALIANT study (VALsartan in Acute myocardial iNfarcTion) [54], which showed that patients with reduced systolic function were at highest risk for sudden cardiac death in the first 30 days after myocardial infarction. Interestingly, an analysis of the MADIT II results, with all the caveats that a subgroup analysis entails, has shown that patients who have recently had a MI do not benefit from an ICD, as opposed to those with old infarcts. The benefit is shown only for remote outside of 18 months that persisted up to 15 years after MI [55]. Although guidelines have adopted a 40-day blanking period from DINAMIT, the optimal timing of ICD implantation remains unknown.

Despite the inclusion of the nonischemic etiologies into class I ICD primary prevention recommendations, not a single trial has demonstrated a statistically significant mortality benefit from ICD in this group. The CAT (Cardiomyopathy Trial) and AMIOVIRT (Amiodarone Versus Implantable Cardioverter Defibrillator Trial) were both terminated prematurely due to futility [56,57]. The largest and only prospective trial of exclusively nonischemic patients was the DEFINITE (Defibrillators in Nonischemic Cardiomyopathy Treatment Evaluation) [58] that showed that the primary end point off all-cause mortality failed to reach statistical significance at 29 months. The low event rates in this study of relatively small simple size may also be attributed to the low usage of amiodarone in the control group, and high equitable rates of β-blockers (85%) and ACE inibitor (95%) as background therapy. The SCD-HeFT (Sudden Cardiac Death Heart FailureTrial) was the largest primary prevention defibrillator trial to date, with a combination of ischemic (52%) and nonischemic (48%) etiologies [59]. Compared with placebo, ICD reduced all-cause mortality from 29% to 22% at 45 months. The 2-year mortality rate was approximately 20%, similar to the MADIT II population. Prespecified subgroup analysis was performed by NYHA class and etiology. Neither ischemic nor nonischemic subgroups met statistical significance. Of note benefit from ICD was see only in NYHA II patients and amiodarone was harmful when compared with placebo in patients with NYHA III. In accordance with statistical dictum, subgroup analysis should be hypothesis generating, rather than leading to practice guidelines [52].

It's also fundamental to emphasize the drug therapy importance. β-Blockers use, which has been demonstrated to reduce arrhythmic and all-cause mortality in the postmyocardial infarction and chronic systolic dysfunction setting, can have an effect on the outcome of ICD trials. First, greater use of β-blockers decrease overall event rates, thereby diminishing the power of a study to demonstrate benefit of ICD therapy if the sample size is not increased. Furthermore, if patients randomized to ICD were disproportionately treated with higher rates of β-blockade, overall benefit seemingly from ICD would bee accentuated. With the exception of SCD-HeFT, trial patients randomized to "control" received antiarrhythmic drug therapy. Although significant differences between randomized groups may be attributed to the superiority of the active treatment tested, the possibility of an inferior performance in the "control" arm, worse than that of placebo, must not be overlooked. The potential for harm from antiarrhythmic therapy has been well documented historically from trials like CAST (Cardiac Arrhythmia Suppression Trial) [39] and SWORD (Survival with Oral D-Sotalol) [60]. The propafenone active treatment arm had to be discontinued in CASH due to a 61% increase in mortality at 11 months [43]. In MADIT, patients in the control group had a 10% higher mortality rate if they were taking amiodarone at 1 month. Antiarrhythmic therapy resulted in a worse prognosis than standard therapy in SCD-HeFT and in MUSTT.

http://dx.doi.org/10.5772/52840

5.2. SCD risk predictors

As ICDs are by design effective in preventing sudden arrhythmic death, their ability to prolong overall survival is associated with the selection of a patient population with sufficiently high incidence of lethal arrhythmias and a sufficiently low incidence of death from all other causes combined. Thus, according to existing evidence, in the modern reperfusion and medical therapy era, a significant survival benefit has been demonstrated only in high-risk patients with ischaemic cardiomyopathy and with an EF of ≤35% usually due to a remote MI [31]. Therefore, substantial reductions in SCD incidence will require effective primary preventive interventions. Since the majority of SCDs occurs in the general population, the primary prevention goal is the identification of high-risk subsets. Numerous invasive and noninvasive techniques have been developed over the years to identify patients at risk for SCD [61-63]. Currently, assessment of left ventricular EF is commonly used to identify high-risk patients and to guide primary prevention of SCD [49]. EF is simple to evaluate, and has been a qualifying criterion of all the primary prevention trials. Concerns have been raised that EF is unlikely to be sufficient for effective SCD risk prediction, because it lacks both sensitivity and specificity [10]. Risk stratification for sudden cardiac death is an active field of investigation. Because of the dire consequences of the first clinical episode, there is a high degree of motivation in the medical community and patient community to identify individuals at risk for sudden cardiac death before its first manifestation. The Cardiac Arrhythmias and Risk Stratification after Acute Myocardial Infarction (CARISMA) study [64] performed a comprehensive analysis of a number of well-accepted risk markers for sudden cardiac death and compared them to each other. The findings are instructive, particularly in relation to the kind of information we can expect from any one of these risk stratification tests. To illustrate this concept, a new hypothetical risk stratification test will be proposed. The new test, a coin toss, will indicate that a patient is at high risk if the coin lands on "heads" and that a patient is at low risk if the coin lands on "tails." Intuitively, this test should provide absolutely no risk stratification. The positive and negative predictive values of this test are calculated in the CARISMA population. The positive predictive value of a coin toss is 8.3%; and the negative predictive value is 92.3%. As would be expected, the sensitivity and specificity of the coin toss approximate 50%. The coin toss performs minimally less well than left ventricular EF, the clinical parameter that is predominantly relied upon for risk stratification [65]. The same findings have been described in the Alternans Before Cardioverter Defibrillator (ABCD) Trial [66] which has repeated the coin toss experiment. Clinical decision-making is a complex process. Particularly when it comes to risk stratification for sudden cardiac death, it involves more than just a simple interpretation of a single test and implementation of therapy based on a single test. Yet, there are several important lessons from the coin toss experiment. When the overall incidence of events is low in the population (8.0% in CARISMA and 11.5% in ABCD), the negative predictive value of any test, even a coin toss, will be very high. This is because the number of true negatives far outweighs the number of false negatives. Although it is desirable to have a simple test to identify risk for sudden cardiac death, it can be seen that even with the use of currently available tests known to identify increased risk for sudden cardiac death, the ability to use these tests to make individual decisions is limited [67]. One option to improve risk stratification is to find some test that provides better discrimination. Taken together, the available experience suggests that multiple risk markers used in combination may provide a more robust prediction of events, which is not surprising when one considers the complexity and diversity of electro-anatomic substrates that underlie SCD.

The low predictive power of the EF in the community is well documented: less than a third off all SCD cases have severely decreased EF (≤ 35%) that would have qualified them as candidates for ICD therapy [68]. Conversely, an analysis of data from the MUSTT has shown that patients whose only risk factor is EF of ≤ 30%, and would qualify for ICD therapy according to current guidelines, may have a predicted 2-year arrhythmic death risk of <5% [69]. Analysis of the MADIT II patients also indicates that the benefit of the ICD in the low EF population may not be uniform [50]. Depending on the presence of other risk factors, patients with EF from 30 to 40% may have total mortality and sudden death risks that exceed those of some patients with EF of ≤ 30% [69].

5.3. Comorbidity

Noncardiac comorbidity, such as diabetes mellitus, cerebrovasular disease, chronic obstructive pulmonary disease, and advanced renal failure, plays a pivotal role in the prognosis of a patient with arrhythmias. Despite the advances in medical therapy, the prognosis of heart failure patients is poor. The majority of heart failure patients has more than one condition affecting their health state. An increasing number of noncardiac comorbidities has the potential to blunt or negate the benefit of ICD therapy due to competing risks for death [52]. The potential futility of ICD efficacy in patients with chronic and end-stage renal disease has been suggested by multiple retrospective cohort analyses [70-73]. The Charlson comorbidity index (CCI) is widely used as an adjustment variable in prognostic models [74]. The index is based on comorbid conditions and cardiovascular risk factors of known prognostic value with varying assigned weights. A recent study showed that patients with a high comorbidity burden, defined as an age-adjusted CCI ≥ 5, had an increased risk for mortality, independent from the prevention indication [4]. The majority of patients who died prior to appropriate ICD therapy had a primary prevention indication. Despite the effectiveness of terminating ventricular tachyarrhythmias by the ICD, competing non-cardiac comorbidity is associated with increased mortality [75]. Furthermore the effect of renal function on ICD efficacy was assessed in a retrospective analysis from MADIT II [76]. The study showed exceedingly high mortality rates (2-year Kaplan estimates of death of approximately 40%) in a relatively small subset of MADIT-II patients who had advanced renal dysfunction (estimated glomerular filtration rate [eGFR] <35 mL min^{-1} 1.73 m^{-2}). Death rates in patients with advanced renal disease were dominated by nonarrhythmic mortality. Accordingly, no ICD benefit was shown in MADIT-II patients with eGFR of less than 35 units, whereas the benefit of the ICD was pronounced in patients with eGFR of at least 35 units. These findings suggest caution when considering primary ICD implantation in patients with advanced renal dysfunction [77] and high burden of other noncardiac comorbidity.

http://dx.doi.org/10.5772/52840

5.4. Age

Although elderly patients (> 70 years) remain at highest risk for SCD, comprising more than 65% of 465.000 out-of-hospital deaths in 1999 [78], routine ICD implantation in them is debatable. Patients older than 75 years were underrepresented in the landmark trials, those which have been drawn the guidelines, and patients older than 80 years were specifically excluded in MADIT (mean age 62 ± 9 years). The median age of patients in SCD-HeFT was 61 and patients older than 65 years did not benefit from ICD therapy. The mean age of MADIT II was 64 ± 10, and only 16% of patients enrolled were older than 75 years. A meta-analysis of secondary prevention trials showed that patients older than 75 did not benefit from ICD implantation [79]. More recent meta-analysis of primary prevention trials showed that prophylactic ICD therapy in elderly patients was associated with a nonsignificant reduction in all-cause mortality compared with medical therapy [3]. Single- center ICD registries have demonstrated steep increases in both cardiac e noncardiac mortality in patients older than 75 years [80,81].

Advanced age clearly presents multiple competing risks for death, and age was also a significant independent predictor of mortality in the long-term follow-up of MADIT II. A recent study showed that age and GFR are the only indipendent predictors of survival in patients ≥ 80 years old, whereas ICD do not appear to influence the overall survival [82]. Of note, in none of the ICD recipients followed in this study there were any true instances of documented ventricular fibrillation, which adds to the evidence that ICDs are unlike to influence survival in this patient population and is consistent with previous reports [83]. A consistent finding, however, is that older patients have an increased risk of death and an altered profile as to their cause of death. Indeed the ratio of SCD to all-cause mortality decreases over age groups such that the lowest ratio is found in patients > 80 years. Thus patients > 80 years old are more like to die from nonarrhythmic or noncardiac causes for which an ICD is not helpful [84]. Other study [80,81] showed that given the increased probability of death from competing causes in elderly patients, patients older than a certain age cease to extract a survival benefit from an ICD. The problem therefore is reduced to identifying this specific age cutoff. Current guidelines do not preclude octogenarians and nonagenarians from receiving ICDs for primary prevention unless they have < 1-year life expectancy [1]. In primary prevention ICD trials, which constitute the basis for current clinical practice, more than 50% of enrolled patients were younger than 60 years [49,53,58,59,85]. In real-world practice, nearly 70% of ICDs are implanted in patients older than 60 years, and more than 40% are implanted in patients older than 70 years [83]. A primary prevention indication accounts for two thirds of cases in which such devices are used. The real-world extrapolation of data has resulted in 1 out of 6 Medicare ICD implants in patients older than 80 years, with a mean age of 70. The ACT registry (Advancements in ICD Therapy) showed that more than 40% of patients undergoing primary prevention ICD implantation were older than 70 years, with 12% older than 80 [83]. In light of this evidence and given of the cost and the potential risks associated with ICD implantation, the benefit of ICD therapy in the elderly are not well established. Of note, the benefit of cardiac resynchronization therapy (CRT), which reduces predominantly nonarrhythmic mortality (for example, heart failure mortality), seems consistent across different age groups. Subgroup analyses of CRT trials have reported a similar degree of CRT benefit in elderly and younger patients [86-88]. Taken together, these findings support that CRT alone may be the best device therapy in elderly persons with severe left ventricular dysfunction.

This upward drift in age representation in the real world not substantiated by trial data is concerning, not only on scientific grounds but from an ethic and philosophic viewpoint.

5.5. Gender

Different studies suggest that the incidences of various types of cardiac arrhythmia are different for women and men, although in many cases we still do not know why this should be. Two principle mechanisms have been proposed to explain these differences between the sexes differential: hormonal effects on the expression or function of ion channels or, conversely, differences in autonomic tone. It is also possible that a combination of these 2 mechanisms may be involved. A combined mechanism would lead to greater sympathetic activity and a lower baroreflex response in men of any age as well as to more pronounced parasympathetic or vagal activity in women. Experimental animal models studies, that used ovariectomized females treated with different gonadal steroids, suggest that the gonadal steroids are responsible for the differences, thanks to their effects on the ion channels of the cell membrane. These differences between sexes have some clinical implications, particularly for the therapeutic approach and clinical treatment of arrhythmias in women [89]. Differences in ventricular tachycardia and sudden death between the sexes were also reported in the Framingham study [90]. After a follow-up of 26 years, the incidence of sudden death increased with the age of the population, with a predominance in men in all age groups and an overall ratio in the incidence of approximately 3:1 compared to woman. This difference was explained by the epidemiology of the heart disease (in women, it appears 10 years to 20 years later). An analysis of survival in the VALIANT study, conducted in 14.703 patients with heart failure and ventricular dysfunction after myocardial infarction, revealed that 1067 cases of sudden death were reported during follow-up. Of these, 67% occurred in men and 33% in women [91]. The presence of gender differences in sudden cardiac death substrates and mechanisms has been reported also in epidemiological studies evaluating out-of-hospital cardiac arrest, which showed that women present more commonly with asystole and pulseless electrical activity, whereas men usually have ventricular tachycardia and ventricular fibrillation [92]. Subgroup analysis in several primary prevention trials revealed that the reduction of overall mortality achieved by ICD was more pronounced in male patients and it did not reach statistically significant levels in women [49,58,59]. In addition, a meta-analysis of 4 major primary prevention trials [93] found no mortality benefit of ICDs in women. After prophylactic ICD implantation, the mortality reduce significantly in men (HR 0,67, 95% CI 0,58-0,78, $p<0{,}001$), whereas in women the mortality reduction was inconclusive (HR 0,78, 95% CI 0,57-1,05, $p=0{,}1$) [94]. These data confirm that EF is not a reliable sudden death risk factor in women. At variance with ICD studies subgroup analyses of CRT trials suggest

http://dx.doi.org/10.5772/52840

that women may have a better response to CRT, with significantly lower incidence of the combined endpoint of first heart failure hospitalization or death, better degree of left ventricular reverse remodeling [88, 95-97].

6. Conclusions

The existing evidence does not support recommendations for ICD implantation by current guidelines on several occasions. We may over treat certain patients. As current guidelines have been broadened to include lower-risks groups with lower event rates, the cost-effectiveness of ICD therapy has become even less favorable. Implantable cardioverter-defibrillators are life-saving in high-risk population that, however, cannot be defined simply by the EF. The ICD does not confer immortality. It is most likely to result in meaningful prolongation of life in patients who are at high risk for lethal arrhythmias but low risk of death from hemodynamic failure or other organ system disease [98]. Further studies are necessary for identifying the most appropriately "at-risk" population for ICD therapies and the guidelines should be re-evaluated and updated. Serious comorbidities that limit the life expectancy of the patient, as well as gender and age should also be taken into account. The adoption of strict criteria for ICD implantation is a necessary step toward a rational use of our limited resources, particularly in an era of economic uncertainty and financial crises [31]. Finally, the ICD implantation should be preceded by a careful analysis of risk/benefit balance, shared with the patient and his family. Comunication with these patients focused on a horizon of 5 years, during which for every 100 patients receiving devices, approximately 30 patients are predicted to die with or without an ICD, while 7 to 8 lives may be saved with the ICD. These estimates are presented in the context of adverse events, including unnecessary shocks, and the possibility that circumstances may arise for which the defibrillator may be inactivated to allow natural death [99]. Considerations of an individual's age comordibity, and remaining life expectancy have a vital place not only in decision-making regarding expensive and invasive procedures such as ICD implantation, but also for "routine" health screenings. Many questions still remain open.

Author details

Marzia Giaccardi[1], Andrea Colella[2], Giovanni Maria Santoro[1], Alfredo Zuppiroli[1] and Gian Franco Gensini[2]

1 Cardiology Department ASL 10, Florence, Italy

2 Heart and Vessels Department AOU Careggi, University of Florence, Italy

References

[1] Epstein AE, Di Marco JP, Ellenbogen KA, et al. ACC/AHA/HRS 2008 Guidelines for Device-Based Therapy of Cardiac Rhythm Abnormalities: a report of the American College of Cardiology/American Heart Association Task Force on Practice Guidelines (Writing Committee to Revise the ACC/AHA/NASPE 2002 Guideline Update for Implantation of Cardiac Pacemakers and Antiarrhythmia Devices): developed in collaboration with the American Association for Thoracic Surgery and Society of Thoracic Surgeons. Circulation 2008;117: e350–e408.

[2] Santangeli P, Di Biase L, Perlagonio G, et al. Outcome of invasive electrophysiological procedures and gender: Are Males ad Females the same? J CardiovascElectrophysiol 2011; 22:605-612.

[3] Santangeli P, Di Biase L, Dello Russo A, et al. Meta-analysis: Age and effectinevess of prophylactic implantable cardioverter- defibrillators. Ann Intern Med 2010;153:592-599.

[4] Theuns DAMJ, Schaer BA, Soliman OI, et al. The prognosis of implantable defibrillator patients treated with cardiac resynchronization therapy: comorbidity burden as predictor of mortality. Europace 2011;13:62-69.

[5] U.S. Dept. of Veterans Affairs, http://www.va.gov/trm/TRMGlossaryPage.asp.

[6] Myerburg RJ, Reddy V, Castellanos A. Indications for Implantable Cardioverter-Defibrillators Based on Evidence and Judgment. JACC 2009;54:747-763.

[7] Tung R, Zimetbaum P, Josephson ME. A Critical Appraisal of Implantable Cardioverter-Defibrillator Therapy for prevention of Sudden Cardiac Death. JACC 2008; 52:1111-1121.

[8] Lopshire JC, Zipes DP. Sudden cardiac death: Better understanding of risks, mechanisms, and treatment. Circulation. 2006;114:1134 –1136.

[9] Zipes DP, Camm AJ, Borggrefe M, et al. ACC/AHA/ESC 2006 guidelines for management of patients with ventricular arrhythmias and the prevention of sudden cardiac death: a report of the American College of Cardiology/American Heart Association task force and the European Society of Cardiology committee for practice guidelines (writing committee to develop guidelines for management of patients with ventricular arrhythmias and the prevention of sudden cardiac death): developed in collaboration with the European Heart Rhythm association and the Heart Rhythm Society. Circulation. 2006;114:e385– e484.

[10] Fishman GI, Chugh S, DiMarco JP, et al. Sudden cardiac death prediction and prevention report from a National Heart, Lung, and Blood Institute and Heart Rhythm Society workshop. Circulation. 2010;122:2335–2348.

[11] Fox CS, Evans JC, Larson MG, et al. Temporal trends in coronary heart disease mortality and sudden cardiac death from 1950 to 1999: the Framingham Heart Study. Circulation. 2004;110:522–527.

[12] Lloyd-Jones D, Adams RJ, Brown TM, et al. American Heart Association Statistics Committee and Stroke Statistics Subcommittee. Heart disease and stroke statistics–2010 update: a report from the American Heart Association. Circulation. 2010;121:e46–e215.

[13] Byrne R, Constant O, Smyth Y, et al. Multiple source surveillance incidence and aetiology of out-of-hospital sudden cardiac death in a rural population in the West of Ireland. Eur Heart J. 2008;29:1418 –1423.

[14] Chugh SS, Jui J, Gunson K, et al. Current burden of sudden cardiac death: multiple source surveillance versus retrospective death certificate-based review in a large U.S. Community. J Am CollCardiol. 2004;44:1268 –1275.

[15] de Vreede-Swagemakers JJ, Gorgels AP, Dubois-Arbouw WI, et al. Out-of-hospital cardiac arrest in the 1990's: a population-based study in the Maastricht area on incidence, characteristics and survival. J Am CollCardiol. 1997;30:1500–1505.

[16] Vaillancourt C, Stiell IG. Cardiac arrest care and emergency medical services in Canada. Can J Cardiol. 2004;20:1081–1090.

[17] Nichol G, Thomas E, Callaway CW, et al. Regional variation in out-of-hospital cardiac arrest incidence and outcome. JAMA. 2008;300:1423–1431.

[18] de Vreede-Swagemakers JJ, Gorgels AP, Dubois-Arbouw WI, et al. Out-of-hospital cardiac arrest in the 1990's: a population-based study in the Maastricht area on incidence, characteristics and survival. J Am Coll Cardiol. 1997;30:1500–1505.

[19] Straus SM, Bleumink GS, Dieleman JP, et al. The incidence of sudden cardiac death in the general population. J ClinEpidemiol. 2004;57:98 –102.

[20] Luu M, Stevenson LW, Baron K, et al. Diverse mechanisms of unexpected cardiac arrest in advanced heart failure. Circulation 1989;80:1675-1680.

[21] Bayes de Luna A, Coumel P, Leclercq JF. Ambulatory sudden cardiac death: mechanisms of production of fatal arrhythmia on the basis of data from 157 cases. Am Heart J. 1989;117:151-159.

[22] Myerburg RJ, Kessler KM, Castellanos A. Sudden cardiac death: structure, function, and time-dependence of risk. Circulation 1992;85(1):I 1-10.

[23] Cobb LA, Fahrenbruch CE, Olsufka M, et al. Changing incidence of out-of-hospital ventricular fibrillation, 1980–2000. JAMA. 2002;288:3008–3013.

[24] Herlitz J, Andersson E, Bång A, et al. Experiences from treatment of out-ofhospital cardiac arrest during 17 years in Go°teborg. Eur Heart J. 2000;21:1251–1258.

[25] Zheng ZJ, Croft JB, Giles WH, et al. Sudden cardiac death in the United States, 1989 to 1998. Circulation. 2001;104:2158 –2163.

[26] Weisfeldt ML, Everson –Stewart S, Sitlani C, et al. Resuscitation Outcomes Consortium Investigators. Ventricular tachyarrhythmias after cardiac arrest in public versus at home. N Engl J Med 2011;364:313-321.

[27] Adabag AS, Therneau TM, Gersh BJ, et al. Sudden death after myocardial infarction. JAMA 2008;300:2022-2029.

[28] Myerburg RJ, Kessler KM, Mallon SM, et al. Life-threatening ventricular arrhythmias in patients with silent myocardial ischemia due to coronary artery spasm. N Engl J Med 1992;326:1451-1455.

[29] Olshausen KV, Stienen U, Schwartz F, et al. Long-term prognostic significance of ventricular arrhythmias in idiopathic dilated-cardiomyopathy. Am J Cardiol 1988;61:146-151.

[30] Hallstrom AP, Ornato JP, Weisfeldt M, et al. Publicaccess defibrillation and survival after out-of-hospital cardiac arrest. N Engl J Med. 2004;351:637– 646.

[31] Katritsis DG, Josephson ME. Sudden cardiac death and implantable cardioverter defibrillators: two modern epidemics? Europace 2012;14:787-794.

[32] Mirowski M, Reid PR, Mower MM, et al. Termination of malignant ventricular arrhythmias with an implanted automatic defibrillator in human beings. N Engl J Med 1980;303:322-344.

[33] Mirowski M, Mower MM, Staewen WS, et al. Standby automatic defibrillator. An approach to prevention of sudden coronary death. Arch Intern Med 1970;126:158–61.

[34] Mirowski M, Mower MM, Mendeloff AI. Implanted standby defibrillators. Circulation 1973;47:1135–1136.

[35] Lown B, Axelrod P. Implanted standby defibrillators. Circulation 1972;46:637–639.

[36] Langer A, Heilman MS, Mower MM, et al. Considerations in the development of the automatic implantable defibrillator. Med Instrum 1976;10:163–167.

[37] Mirowski M, Mower MM, Langer A, et al. A chronically implanted system for automatic defibrillation in active conscious dogs. Experimental model for treatment of sudden death from ventricular fibrillation. Circulation 1978;58:90–94.

[38] The Cardiac Arrhythmia Suppression Trial (CAST) Investigators. Preliminary report: effect of encainide and flecainide on mortality in a randomized trial of arrhythmia suppression after myocardial infarction. N Engl J Med 1989;321:406–412.

[39] Echt DS, Liebson PR, Mitchell LB, et al. Mortality and morbidity in patients receiving encainide, flecainide, or placebo: the Cardiac Arrhythmia Suppression Trial. N Engl J Med 1991;324:781– 788.

[40] Wever EF, Hauer RN, van Capelle FL, et al. Randomized study of implantable defibrillators as first-choice therapy versus conventional strategy in postinfarct sudden death survivors. Circulation 1995;91:2195-2203.

[41] The Antiarrhythmic versus Implantable Defibrillators (AVID) Investigators. A comparison of antiarrhythmic-drug therapy with implantable defibrillators in patients resuscitated from near-fatal ventricular arrhythmias. N Engl J Med 1997;337:1576:1583.

[42] Connoly SJ, Gent M, Roberts RS, et al. Canadian implantable defibrillator study (CIDS): a randomized trial of the implantable cardioverter defibrillator against amiodarone. Circulation 2000;101:1297-1302.

[43] Kuck KH, Cappato R, Siebels J, et al. Randomized comparison of antiarrhythmic drug therapy with implantable defibrillators in patients resuscitated from cardiac arrest: The Cardiac Arrest Study Hamburg (CASH). Circulation 2000;102:748-754.

[44] Domanski MJ, Sakseena S, Epstein AE, et al., for the AVID Investigators. Relative effectiveness of the implantable cardioverterdefibrillator and antiarrhythmic drugs in patients with varying degrees of left ventricular dysfunction who have survived malignant ventricular arrhythmias. AntiarrhythmicsVersus Implantable Defibrillators. J Am CollCardiol 1999;34:1090–1095.

[45] Larsen G, Hallstrom A, McAnulty J. Cost-effectiveness of the implantable cardioverter-defibrillator versus antiarrhythmic drugs in survivors of serious ventricular tachyarrhythmias: results of the Antiarrhythmics Versus Implantable Defibrillators (AVID) economic analysis substudy. Circulation 2002;105:2049–2057.

[46] Connolly SJ, Hallstrom AP, Cappato R, et al. Meta-analysis of the implantable cardioverter defibrillator secondary prevention trials. AVID, CASH and CIDS studies. Antiarrhythmicsvs Implantable Defibrillator study. Cardiac Arrest Study Hamburg. Canadian Implantable Defibrillator Study. Eur Heart J 2000;21:2071–2078.

[47] Moss AJ, Hall WJ, Cannom DS, et al: Improved survival with an implanted defibrillator in patients with coronary disease at high risk for ventricular arrhythmia. Multicenter Automatic Defibrillator Implantation Trial Investigators. N Engl J Med 1996;335:1933-1940.

[48] Buxton AE, Lee KL, Fisher JD, et al. Randomized study of the prevention of sudden death in patients with coronary artery disease. N Engl J Med 1999;341:1882-1890.

[49] Moss AJ, Zareba W, Hall WJ, et al. Prophylactic implantation of a defibrillator in patients with myocardial infarction and reduced ejection fraction. N Engl J Med 2002;346:877-883.

[50] Goldenberg l, Vyas AK, Hall WJ, et al. Risk stratification for primary implantation of a cardioverter defibrillator in patients with ischemic left ventricular dysfunction. J Am CollCardiol 8;51:288-296.

[51] Mitchell, LB; Pineda, EA; Titus, JL; et al. Sudden Death in Patients With Implantable Cardioverter Defibrillators. The Importance of Post-Shock Electromechanical Dissociation. JACC, 2002;39:1323-1328.

[52] Tung R, Josephson ME. Implantable Cardioverter-Defibrillator Therapy for Primary Prevention of Sudden Cardiac Death: An Argument for Restraint. Card ElectrophysiolClin 2009;1:105-116.

[53] Hohnloser SH, Kuck KH, Dorian P, et al. Prophylactic use of an implantable cardioverter-defibrillator after acute myocardial infarction. N Engl J Med 2004;351 : 2481-2488.

[54] Solomon SD, Zelenkofske S, Mclvlurray JJ, et al. Sudden death in patients with myocardial infarction and left ventricular dysfunction, heart failure, or both. N Engl J Med 2005;352;2581-2588.

[55] Wilber DJ, Zareba W, Hall WJ, et al. Time dependence of mortality risk and defibrillator benefit after myocardial infarction. Circulation 2004;109:1082-1084.

[56] Bansch D, Antz M, Boczor S, et al. Primary prevention of sudden cardiac death in idiopathic dilated cardiomyopathy: the Cardiomyopathy Trial (CAT). Circulation 2002;105;1453-1458.

[57] Strickberger SA, Hummel JD, Bartlett TG, et al. Amiodarone versus implantable cardioverter-defibrillator: randomized trial in patients with nonischemic dilated cardiomyopathy and asymptomatic nonsustained ventricular tachycardia- AMIOVIRT. J Am CollCardiol 2003;41;1707-1712.

[58] Kadish A, Dyer A, Daubert JP, et al. Prophylactic defibrillator implantation in patients with nonischemic dilated cardiomyopathy. N Engl J Med 2004;350:2151-2158.

[59] Bardy GH, Lee KL, Mark DB, et al. Amiodarone or an implantable cardioverter-defibrillator for congestive heart failure. N Engl J Med 2005;352:225-237.

[60] Waldo AL, Camm AJ, deRuyter H, et al. Effect of d-sotalol on mortality in patients with left ventricular dysfunction after recent and remote myocardial infarction. The SWORD Investigators. Survival with Oral D-Sotalol. Lancet 1996;348:7-12.

[61] Zipes DP, Wellens HJ. Sudden cardiac death. Circulation. 1998;98:2334–2351.

[62] Bailey JJ, Berson AS, Handelsman H, et al. Utility of current risk stratification tests for predicting major arrhythmic events after myocardial infarction. J Am CollCardiol. 2001;38:1902–1911.

[63] Wilber DJ, Olshansky B, Moran JF, et al. Electrophysiological testing and nonsustained ventricular tachycardia: use and limitations in patients with coronary artery disease and impaired ventricular function. Circulation. 1990;82:350–358.

[64] Huikuri HV, Raatikainen MJ, Moerch-Joergensen R, et al. Prediction of fatal or near-fatal cardiac arrhythmia events in patients with depressed left ventricular function after an acute myocardial infarction. Eur Heart J 2009;30:689-98.

[65] Goldberger JJ. The coin toss: Implications for risk stratification for sudden cardiac death. Am Heart J 2010;160:3-7.

[66] Costantini O, Hohnloser SH, Kirk MM, et al. The ABCD (AlternansBeforeCardiovert-er Defibrillator) Trial: strategies using T-wave alternans to improve efficiency of sudden cardiac death prevention. J Am CollCardiol 2009;53:471-9.

[67] Goldberger JJ. Evidence-based analysis of risk factors for sudden cardiac death. Heart Rhythm 2009;6:S2-S7.

[68] Stecker EC, Vickers C, Waltz J, et al. Populationbased analysis of sudden cardiac death with and without left ventricular systolic dysfunction: two-year findings from the Oregon Sudden Unexpected Death Study. J Am CollCardiol 2006;47:1161–1166.

[69] Buxton AE, Lee KL, Hafley GE, et al. MUSTT Investigators. Limitations of ejection fraction for prediction of sudden death risk in patients with coronary artery disease: lessons from the MUSTT study. J Am CollCardiol 2007;50:1150–7.

[70] Hreybe H, Razak E, Saba S. Effect of end-stage renal failure and hemodialysis on mortality rates in implantable cardioverter defibrillator recipients. Pacing ClinElectrophysiol 2007;30:1091-1095.

[71] Lee DS, Tu JV, Austin PC, et al. Effect of cardiac and noncardiac conditions on survival after defibrillator implantation. J Am CollCardiol 2007;49:2408-2415.

[72] Cuculich PS, Sanchez JM, Kerzner R, et al. Poor prognosis for patients with chronic kidney disease despite ICD therapy for the primary prevention of sudden death. Pacing ClinElectrophysiol 2007:30:207-213.

[73] Bruch C, Sindermann J, Breithardt G, et al. Prevalence and prognostic impact of comorbidities in heart failure patients with implantable cardioverter defibrillator. Europace 2007:9:681-686.

[74] Charlson ME, Pompei P, Ales KL, et al. A new method of classifying prognostic comorbidity in longitudinal studies: development and validation. J Chronic Dis. 1987;40:373–383.

[75] Koller MT, Schaer B, Wolbers M, et al. Death without prior appropriate implantable cardioverter-defibrillator therapy: a competing risk study. Circulation. 2008;117:1918–26.

[76] Goldenberg I, Moss AJ, McNitt S, et al, for the Multicenter Automatic Defibrillator Implantation Trial-II Investigators: Relations among renal function, risk of sudden cardiac death, and benefit of the implanted cardiac defibrillator in patients with ischemic left ventricular dysfunction. Am J Cardiol , 2006;98:485-490.

[77] Goldenberg I, Moss AJ. Implantable Device Therapy. Progress in Cardiovascular Diseases 2008;50:449-474.

[78] Zheng ZJ, Croft JB, Giles WH, et al. State-specific mortality from sudden cardiac death-United States, 1999. MMWR Morb Mortal Wkly Rep 2002;51:123-126.

[79] Healey JS, Hallstrom AP, Kuck KH, et al. Role of the implantable defibrillator among elderly patients with a history of life—threatening ventricular arrhythmias. Eur Heart J 2007;28:1746-1749.

[80] Pellegrini CN, Lee K, Olgin JE, et al. Impact of advanced age on survival in patients with implantable cardioverterclefibrillators. Europace 2008;10:1296-1301.

[81] Panotopoulos PT, Axtell K, Anderson AJ, et al. Efficacy of the implantable cardioverter-defibrillator in the elderly. J Am CollCardiol 1997:29:556-560.

[82] Mezu U, Adelstein E, Jain S, et al. Effectiveness of Implantable Defibrillators in Octogenarians and Nonagenarians for Primary Prevention of Sudden Cardiac Death. Am J Cardiol 2011;108:718-722.

[83] Epstein AE, Kay GN, Plumb VJ, et al. Implantable cardioverter-defibrillator prescription in the elderly. Hearty Rhythm 2009;6:1136-1143.

[84] Krahn AD, Connoly SJ, Roberts RS, et al. Diminishing proportional risk of sudden death with advancing age: implication for prevention of sudden cardiac death. Am Heart J 2004;147:837-840.

[85] Steinbeck G, Andresen D, Seidl K, et al. Defibrillator implantation early after myocardial infarction. N Engl J Med. 2009;361:1427-1436.

[86] Bristow MR, Saxon LA, Boehmer J, et al; Comparison of Medical Therapy, Pacing, and Defibrillation in Heart Failure (COMPANION) Investigators. Cardiac-resynchronization therapy with or without an implantable defibrillator in advanced chronic heart failure. N Engl J Med. 2004;350:2140-2150.

[87] Cleland JG, Daubert JC, Erdmann E, et al; Cardiac Resynchronization-Heart Failure (CARE-HF) Study Investigators. The effect of cardiac resynchronization on morbidity and mortality in heart failure. N Engl J Med. 2005;352:1539-1549.

[88] Moss AJ, Hall WJ, Cannom DS, et al; MADIT-CRT Trial Investigators. Cardiac-resynchronization therapy for the prevention of heart-failure events. N Engl J Med. 2009;361:1329-1338.

[89] Bernal O, Moro C. Cardiac Arrhythmias in Women. Rev EspCardiol 2006;59:609–618.

[90] Kannel WB, Wilson PW, d'Agostino RB, et al. Sudden coronary death in women. Am Heart J 1998;136:205-212.

[91] Solomon SD, Zelenkofske S, McMurray JV, et al. Sudden death in patients with myocardial infarction and left ventricular dysfunction, heart failure or both. N Engl J Med 2005;352:2581-2588.

[92] Wigginton JG, Pepe PE, Bedolla JP, et al. Sex related differences in the presentation and outcome of out-of-hospital cardiopulmonary arrest: A multiyear, prospective, population-based study. Crit Care Med 2002;30:S131-S136.

[93] Ghanbari H, Dalloul G, Hasan R, et al. Effectiveness of implantable cardioverter-defibrillators for the primary prevention of sudden cardiac death in women with ad-

vanced heart failure: a meta-analysis of randomized controlled trials. Arch Intern Med 2009;169:1500–1506.

[94] Santangeli P, Pelargonio G, Dello Russo A, et al. Gender differences in clinical outcome and primary prevention defibrillator benefit in patients with severe left ventricular dysfunction: A systematic review and meta-analysis. Heart Rhythm 2010;7:876-882.

[95] Lilli A, Ricciardi G, Porciani MC, et al. Gender related differences in left ventricular reverse remodeling. Pacing ClinElectrophysiol 2007;30:1349-1355.

[96] Woo GW, Petersen-Stejskal S, Johnson JW, et al. Ventricular reverse remodeling and 6-month outcomes in patients receiving cardiac resynchronization therapy: Analysis of the MIRACLE study. J Interv Card Electrophysiol 2005;12:107-113.

[97] Di Biase L, Auricchio A, Sorgente A, et al. The magnitude of reverse remodelling irrespective of aetiology predicts outcome of heart failure patients treated with cardiac resynchronization therapy. Eur Heart J 2008;29:2497-2505.

[98] Josephson M, Wellens HJ. Implantable defibrillators and sudden cardiac death. Circulation 2004;109:2685-2691.

[99] Stevenson LW, Desai AS. Selecting patients for discussion of the ICD as primary prevention for sudden death in heart failure. Journal of Cardiac Failure 2006;12:407-412.

Chapter 5

Long-Term Benefit and Challenges of Implantable Cardioverter Defibrillator Therapy

Damir Erkapic and Tamas Bauernfeind

Additional information is available at the end of the chapter

http://dx.doi.org/10.5772/52325

1. Introduction

The implantable cardioverter defibrillator (ICD) is currently considered the first therapy option to protect patients from life-threatening ventricular arrhythmias. Several randomized studies demonstrated a reduction in total mortality of up to 55% and a reduction in arrhythmogenic mortality of up to 76% in ICD recipients.[1-7] Within a time frame of about 20 years, indications for ICD have evolved from a restricted "last resort therapy" to a secondary and primary preventive therapy. According to HRS/EHRA Expert Consensus on the Monitoring of Cardiovascular Implantable Electronic Devices [8], incidence of ICD implantation in the US and Europe in 2007 was 235,000 and 88,000, respectively, with a upward trend.

Moreover, prevention of sudden cardiac death (SCD) through the ICD is generally considered to represent a therapy, which will be needed for the rest of the patient's life. However, regarding ICD cost-effectiveness as well as the potential risks of ICD therapy and subsequent generator changes the question rises if patients without any adequate ICD intervention during the lifespan of their index ICD really need further ICD protection. Therefore, the question whether or not to replace an ICD generator at the time of battery depletion is of great importance not only for the affected patients but also for their physicians and cost carriers.

This chapter is aimed to give an overview about the currently published data on long-term benefit of ICD therapy based on the incidence of adequate ICD therapy and in the ratio of potentially serious complications.

2. Long-term benefit of ICD therapy

2.1. Secondary prevention trials

Already in 1991, Tchou et al.[9] reported in a single center cohort of 184 patients who received an ICD between 1982 and 1989 (84% with ventricular fibrillation (VF) or sustained ventricular tachycardia (VT), 9% with non-sustained VT (NSVT) and 6% with pre-/syncope) that the actual risk of receiving an adequate shock by the fifth year after implantation was 69%, with an observed bimodal distribution: high within first year, and rise after four years. Occurrence of adequate ICD shock was defined as electrocardiographic documentation (ECG) of sustained VT at the time of shock or if it was preceded by sudden onset of severe presyncopal symptoms or syncope.

Grimm et al.[10] investigated ICD therapy episodes which occurred for the first time in patients who did not require such therapy prior to generator change. This was a prospective single center study enrolling 26 secondary prevention patients (77% with cardiac arrest and 23 with sustained VT) who received their second ICD device 30±9 months after initial ICD implantation. Notably, at that time patients had epicardial electrodes, and only a single patient had an ICD generator with the option to memorize endocardialelectrograms. Adequate shocks were defined as spontaneous ICD discharges preceded by severe symptoms like presyncope or syncope or documentation of VT/VF by Holter or telemetry monitoring or stored ECG by ICD. During a mean follow-up period of 21±9 months after ICD generator replacement, ICD therapy was reported in 13 of 26 patients (50%), classified as adequate in 9 patients (35%).

Dürsch et al.[11] aimed to evaluate retrospectively the necessity of the replacement of ICD generators in patients without any adequate, spontaneous ventricular arrhythmia episode during the life-time of the first implanted device. This study, reported in 1998, compared 62 secondary prevention patients (mean follow-up 51 ± 14 months) with an elective generator replacement due to battery depletion with 151 ICD patients without replacement (follow-up 16.5 ± 11 months). There was a preponderance of male patients (>80%) with a mean left ventricular ejection fraction (LVEF) of 31% in both groups. In contrast to the study of Grimm et al. 86% of patients had transveonusendocardial ICD electrodes and 95% of devices (following generator exchange) had the option to memorize endocardial cardiograms. At that time most of the ICD systems had the capability of antitachycardiac pacing (ATP) prior to ICD shock delivery. For the total patient group there was a 5 year event-free probability of 23%, and no differences were found between the two groups. Subanalysis of the replacement group patients revealed no difference in the probability of adequate ICD therapy occurrence prior to or after the replacement of the pulse generator. Notably, in 6 of the 62 (10%) patients, the first adequate ICD therapy was documented after generator replacement.

Tandri et al.[12] reported in 2006 a single center ICD registry of 1382 patients, who received their first ICD between 1980 and 2003 (76% men, LVEF 33 ± 11%) with mainly secondary prevention indication (77%). In 787 (57%) of these patients ICD therapy informations were available. Adequate ICD therapy was determined based either on the ICD memory or for ICDs without ECG storage capability on the symptoms that preceded

http://dx.doi.org/10.5772/52325

the shock. During a mean follow-up of 70 ± 51 months 53% of the patients received adequate ICD therapy, two thirds of them within the first year of implantation. Out of 127 patients (16%) without adequate ICD therapy within 5 years following the index generator implantation, 8%, 20% and 24% of patients experienced adequate ICD therapy after 6, 10 and 15 years of follow-up, respectively.

Data from another single center ICD registry were reported by Koller et al. in 2008.[13] This registry comprised data of 442 patients with predominantly secondary prevention (59%) with ischemic (76%) or dilated cardiomyopathy (24%) with a median follow-up of 3.6 years (max 12.7 years). Adequate ICD therapy of ventricular arrhythmias stored by intracardiacelectrograms had to be confirmed by an experienced electrophysiologist. The cumulative incidence of any adequate ICD therapy was 52% during a 7-year observation period with a twofold higher risk for patients with secondary prevention compared to primary prevention. Patients without former adequate ICD therapy within 6 years after the first ICD implantation had an observed risk of only 6% for adequate ICD intervention in the following 2 years. Notably, only 35 patients (8%) had follow-up longer than 6 year.

The long-term follow-up of the Leiden Out-of-Hospital Cardiac Arrest Trial (LOHCAT)[14] was the first prospective single center observational study to assess the rate of mortality and risk of adequate ICD therapy in patients with secondary prevention. A total of 456 patients (86% males, mean LVEF 35±14%) with ischemic heart disease and secondary prevention indication were followed for 54±35 months after ICD implantation. Adequate ICD therapy was checked by printouts of the ICD memory. During follow-up 22% of the patients died. The cumulative incidence of adequate ICD therapy at 1, 5, and 8 years was 24, 52 and 61%, respectively. Independent factors for higher risk of adequate ICD intervention were previous VT, history of AF, wide QRS and poor LVEF. No predictive factors for the absence of ventricular arrhythmia could be identified. Of the 456 patients, 167 (37%) outlived the life-span of their index ICD and got generator replacement. No data were reported concerning how many of these patients had no former adequate ICD therapy and/or received the first adequate ICD Therapy after generator replacement.

The INcidence free SUrvival after ICD Replacement (INSURE)[15] trial was the first prospective multicenter observational study to evaluate the risk of adequate ATP and/or ICD shock delivery after elective ICD replacement. A total of 510 unselected ICD-patients with (48%) and without (52%) former adequate ICD therapy were enrolled in 29 germancenters from 2002 until 2007 after an average life-span of their first ICD generator of 62±18 months. After device replacement patients were followed every 3 to 6 months (mean follow-up 22±16 months) until occurrence of an adequate ICD therapy (stored by intracardiacelectrograms and confirmed by an adjudication committee consisting of three experienced electrophysiologists), death, second generator replacement or until common study termination endpoint. The vast majority (86%) of patients had initially been implanted for secondary prevention of SCD. The cumulative rates of adequate ICD interventions after one, two and three years following generator replacement were 32.4%, 41.3% and 48.1% in patients with former adequate ICD therapy and 10.6%, 17.6% and 21.4% in patients without former adequate ICD therapy, respectively (HR 3.08, CI: 2.15-4.39, $p < 0.001$) (Figure 2). In patients without former adequate ICD interventions, only advanced NYHA stages were associated with higher risk of adequate ICD interventions. However, no predictive factors for lower probability of ICD therapy could be identified in this group.

Author / Study	Year	N	Age (mean y)	Male (%)	LVEF (mean%)	ICM (%)	NICM (%)	CAD (%)	no HD (%)
Tchou et al.	1991	184	61±11	81	37±14	n.r.	17	81	3
Grimm et al.	1993	26	56±15	73	38±15	n.r.	20	65	15
Dürsch et al.	1998	62	58±11	89	31±9	34		66	-
Tandri et al.	2006	1382	62±11	76	33±11	72	28	70	-
Koller et al.	2008	442	63	89	30	76	24	76	-
Borleffs et al.	2008	456	65	86	35±14	100	-	100	-
Van Welsenes et al.	2011	832	63±13	82	37±15	73	n.r.	73	n.r.
Erkapic et al.	2012	510	65±10	83	39±16	37	25	71	38

LVEF: left ventricular ejection fraction; **ICM**: ischemic cardiomyopathy; **NICM**: non-ischemic cardiomyopathy; **CAD**: coronary artery disease; **no HD**: no heart disease. **n.r.**: not reported

Table 1. Baseline characteristics of patients in secondary prevention trials with long-term follow-up

Author / Study	Kind of study	FU prior 1. ICD replacement (mean months)	FU after 1. ICD replacement (mean months)	Overall FU (mean months)	First adequate ICD therapy
Tchou et al.	retro. s.c.	24±19	-	-	69% within 5y
Grimm et al.	pros. s.c.	30±9	21±19	-	35% within 6y
Dürsch et al.	retro. s.c.	-	-	50±14	77% within 5 y (thereof 10% after ICD replacement)
Tandri et al.	retro. s.c.	70±51	46±34	-	53% within 5 y (additional 24% after ICD replacement)
Koller et al.	retro. s.c.	-	-	43	52% within 7 y
Borleffs et al.	pros. s.c.	-	-	54±35	61% within 8 y
Van Welsenes et al.	retro. s.c.	41±34	-	-	51% within 5 y
Erkapic et al.	pros. m.c.	62±18	22±16	-	21% within 3 y after ICD replacement

Retro s.c.: retrospective single center-study; **pros. s.c.:** prospective single center-study; **pros. m.c.:** prospective multi-center study; **FU:** follow-up; **y:** years.

Table 2. Incidence of adequate ICD therapy according to follow-up time in secondary prevention trials

2.2. Primary prevention trials

The first trial which tried to provide data on the long-term benefit of ICD therapy in primary prevention patients was published in 2008 by Alsheikh-Ali.[16] Patients with prior myocardial infarction and LVEF ≤35% who received ICD for primary prevention between 1995 and 2005 formed the basis of this retrospective single center analysis. Of 525 predominantly male patients, 115 (22%) received adequate ICD therapy during a mean follow-up of 24 months. Patients who survived more than 5 years after ICD implantation without adequate therapy, the incidence of adequate ICD intervention was 6% after 7 years of follow-up. These observations were in accordance to the data of Koller et al. who reported the same incidence for patients with secondary prevention 7 years after ICD implantation. However, in both studies only 6-8% of patients had follow-up longer than 6 years after first ICD implantation. No predictive factors for a lower probability of ICD therapy could be identified in both studies.

The extended 8-year follow-up study of the Multicenter Automatic Defibrillator Implantation (MADIT) IITrial was published in 2010.[17] Post-trial mortality data for all study participants were obtained from the enrolling centers through hospital records and death registries from 2001 until 2009. One-thousand-twenty study patients who survived to trial closure of MADIT II formed the basis of this study. The primary endpoint was the occurrence of all-cause mortality during a median follow-up of 7.6 years. Patients who were treated with an ICD showed a significant lower risk of death (34%) compared with non-ICD patients. The evident benefit of ICD therapy continued even in the long-term follow-up of up to 8 years, but only for patients with single chamber ICD. Patients with a dual chamber ICD (programmed to active DDD-pacing regardless of conduction abnormalities) and more advanced NYHA class (≥ II) at enrolment, experienced a late increase in mortality due to unnecessary right ventricular pacing leading to progressive heart failure. This observation underlines previous reported data.[18] Regarding the long-term benefit due to adequate ICD therapy in the extended MADIT II trial, the cumulative probability of adequate ICD intervention during 8 years of follow-up was 68%. However, complete information of ICD interrogation during long term follow-up was only available in 109 patients (10,7%) during the post-trial period.

Author / Study	Year	N	Age (mean y)	Male (%)	LVEF (mean%)	ICM (%)	NICM (%)	CAD (%)
Alsheikh-Ali et al.	2008	525	67±11	81	23±7	100	-	100
Goldenberg et al.	2010	630	64±11	85	≤35	100	-	100
Van Welsenes et al.	2011	1302	63±11	80	29±12	68	32	68
Van Welsenes et al.	2011	114	61±11	80	26±9	59	41	59

LVEF: left ventricular ejection fraction; **ICM**: ischemic cardiomyopathy; **NICM**: non-ischemic cardiomyopathy; **CAD**: coronary artery disease.

Table 3. Baseline characteristics of patients in primary prevention trials with long-term follow-up

Author / Study	Kind ofstudy	FU prior 1. ICD replacement (mean months)	FU after 1. ICD replacement (mean months)	Overall FU (mean months)	First adequate ICD therapy
Alsheikh-Ali et al.	retro. s.c.	24±0.4	-	-	22% within 7y
Goldenberg et al.	retro. m.c.	18 (10-30)	n.r.	91 (42-108)	68% within 8y
Van Welsenes et al.	retro. s.c.	41±34	-	-	37% within 5 y
Van Welsenes et al.	retro. s.c.	71±24	25±21	-	14% within 3 y after ICD replacement

retros.c.: retrospective single center-study; retro. **m.c.**: retrospective multi-center study; **FU:** follow-up; **y:** years.

Table 4. Incidence of adequate ICD therapy according to follow-up time in primary prevention trials

Van Welsenes et al. published two reports in 2011 on long-term follow-up data of a single center registry of patients with primary and secondary prevention. In the first publication[19]they reported all-cause mortality and incidence of adequate ICD therapies in patients with primary (61%) and secondary (39%) prevention during the lifetime of the first implanted ICD. The mean follow-up was 3.4±2.8 years. The cumulative 5-year incidence of mortality was 25% for primary and 23% for secondary prevention, without reaching statistifical significance between the two groups. The cumulative 5-year incidence of adequate ICD therapy (each episode had to be confirmed by a trained electrophysiologist by regarding the ICD memory/printouts) was 37% for primary and 51% for secondary prevention patients (Figure 1).

The second puplication[20] comprised data of 114 patients with exclusively primary prevention who did not receive adequate therapy during the lifetime of their first ICD generator. The data were released from the same single center registry and were the first on the topic: "long-term benefit of ICD-therapy after elective device replacement in primary prevention patiens". The single center cohort consisted of mainly ischemic heart disease patients (80% male, mean age 61±11 years) with a mean LVEF of 26%. After an average life-span of their first ICD generator of 71±24 months the patients were followed after elective device replacement for 25±21 months. The cumulative event rate for adequate ICD intervention after replacement increased continuously from 7% after one, 9% after two, to 14% after 3 years (Figure 3).

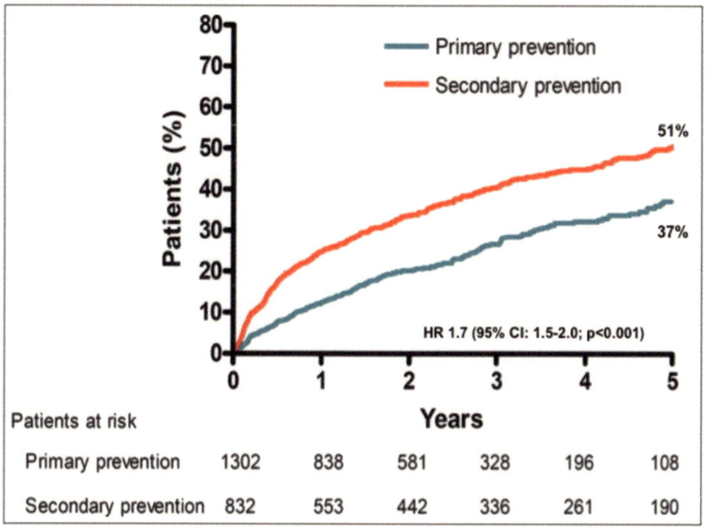

Figure 1. Cumulative incidence of adequate ICD therapies prior elective generator replacement in patients with primary and secondary prevention

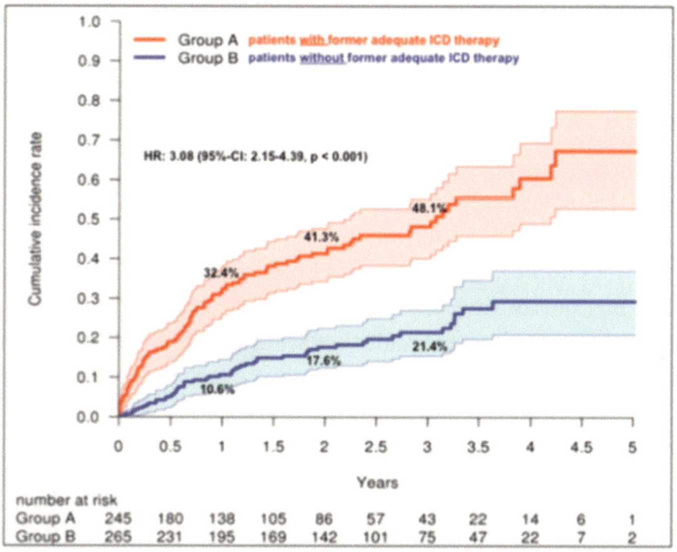

Figure 2. Cumulative incidence of first adequate ICD therapies (with confidence intervals) after elective device replacement in patients with secondary prevention

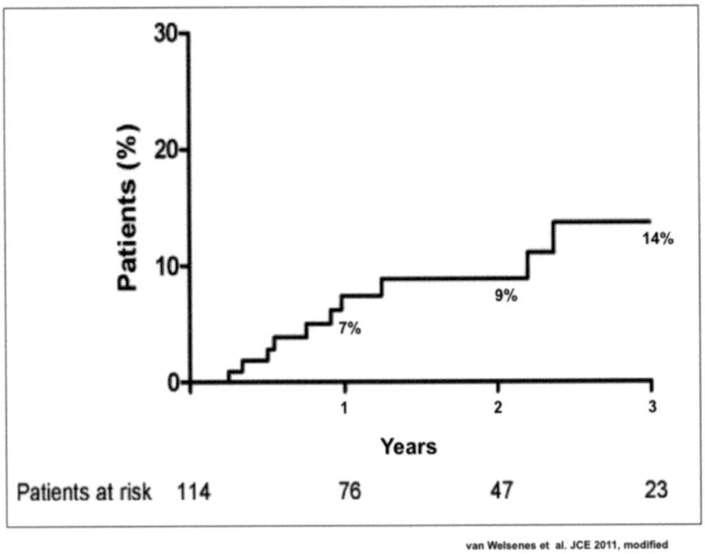

Figure 3. Cumulative incidence of first adequate ICD therapies after elective device replacement in patients with primary prevention without prior adequate ICD therapy

3. Challenges of long term ICD therapy

The long-term benefit of ICD therapy has to be evaluated compared to the ratio of potentially serious complications.

A number of important medical and technological advances in ICD therapies have been made in the last years which helped to reduce the interventional stress for patients and to improve their daily safety[14-19]: the introduction of transvenousendocardial leads, subpectoral or subfascial implantation of smaller and more powerful ICD devices, introduction of diagnostic tools as e.g. monitoring of intrathoracic fluid status, ST segment changes as well as the introduction of remote home monitoring systems. However, ICD therapy is still associated with significant morbidity and some mortality, especially in long-term follow up.

3.1. Lead failure

One of the major risks of long-term ICD therapy is lead failure, mostly presented as lead fracture or insulation defect. The annual lead failure rate increases with time and reaches 20% in 10-year old leads.[20] Mechanical stress on leads is the most frequent cause for lead failure and can be reduced by avoiding the medial subclavian puncture during ICD implantation (preferred approach is through the cephalic vein or lateral subclavian puncture) and by avoiding subpectoral device implantation (preferred subfascial pocket, if possible). However, careful evaluation required, for the latter may result in pocket complications necessitating revision operations.

http://dx.doi.org/10.5772/52325

With the introduction of leads with multilumen design in 1997, lead survival curves initially improved but were still limited due to missing long-lasting insulation material. Silicon which is most often used for lead insulation has a good biocompatibility and flexibility, has a high friction resistance but prone to abrasion of lead insulation material. Even today in a certain type of ICD lead (RIATA®, SJM, Sylmar, CA) with silicon insulation (removed 2010 from distribution), time-dependent incidence of lead failure of 8-33% were reported.[21-24] The same lead model with a silicone-polyurethane copolymer (Optim™, SJM, Sylmar, CA) showed no increased incidence of lead failure, suggesting a better abrasion resistance.[22,25]

Apart from lead insulation material, very small diameter of the ICD lead seemed to be a further risk factor of lead failure.[26] The 6.6 Sprint fidelis® lead (Medtronic, Inc., Minneapolis, MN) is prone to increased chance of lead fracture due to most likely less stress resistance. In 2008 this high-voltage ICD-lead was removed from the market. Actually, incidence of lead failure of 17% at 5 years of follow-up is reported for this lead.[27] Therefore, implanted Sprint fidelis and several Riata lead models should be carefully examined at the time of generator replacement.

3.2. Inadequate ICD therapy

Inadequate ICD therapy is a significant clinical issue. In literature it`s reported that 12-30% of ICD patients receive inadequate ICD therapies, mainly caused by supraventricular tachycardias, T-wave oversensing and lead failure.[28-30] Such unnecessary ICD therapies are associated with increase of posttraumatic disorders as depression and anxiety.[31]It is still a matter of debate, if aside of morbidity, inadequate ICD shocks also have worse impact on the outcome of ICD patients.[30,32] However, it is our firm conviction, that the number of unnecessary ICD therapies triggered by SVTs can be considerably reduced by adequate ICD programming by an experienced physician. Furthermore, newer ICD algorithms reduced inadequate ICD therapy triggered by T-wave oversensing by 97% while maintaining 100% sensitivity for detection of true ventricular arrhythmia.[33]The safety, efficacy and performance of further new ICD discrimination algorithms is actually evaluated in a prospective multi-center trial.[34]

Since the introduction of the Lead Integrity Alert™ (LIA) by Medtronic in 2008, inadequate ICD therapies decreased by up to 50% in patients with fractured Sprint fidelis leads.[35,36] Moreover, it has been reported that this algorithm has the potential to early detect lead failure of the affected Riata family®.[37]

3.3. Risk of ICD generator replacement

Device replacement is associated with significant morbidity and some mortality. Data from a multicenter prospective registry of 1081 ICD patients who underwent device replacement (79% males, mean age 64±13 years) showed a complication rate of 4.3%. Major complications were observed in 2,6%, mostly infections or lead revisions. On multivariate analysis the presence of advanced Canadian Cardiovascular Society angina class (CCS ≥2), advanced NYHA stages (≥III), complex device systems (especially cardiac resynchronization systems), any previous surgery, and low operator procedure volume were predictive factors for overall complication after ICD replacement. Any complication was associated with an increased risk of mortality at 45, 90, and 180 days after device replacement with a HR of 8.58, 9.91 and 4.06, respectively (p=0.005 to 0.069).

It is strongly recommended that risks for complications after ICD replacement should not be underestimated. Even if generator replacement is technically less challenging than a new device implantation, it should be preferably performed by experienced operators.

4. Summary/Conclusion

The currently available literature reveals that patients with adequate ICD therapy prior elective ICD replacement have approximately 3-fold higher risk to receive adequate ICD intervention thereafter compared to patients without prior adequate ICD therapy. However, a significant number of patients without adequate ICD therapy prior elective device replacement will receive adequate ICD intervention thereafter too. In this patient population it is expected that approximately every 5th with secondary and every 7th with primary prevention will receive adequate ICD therapy within 3 years following elective device replacement. Patients who present at poor clinical status with more advanced stages of heart failure, especially with advanced NYHA classes (≥2), as well as patients with secondary prevention indication are at higher risk for adequate ICD therapy in long-term follow-up. No predictive factors for lower probability of ICD therapy could be identified for patients without adequate ICD therapy prior device replacement. Hence, ICD replacement appears still necessary in these patients. Risks of ICD therapy should not be underestimated but the weight of evidence for long-term benefit based on the incidence of ventricular arrhythmias with subsequent adequate ICD therapy supports the continuing use of ICD therapy for patients with adequate ICD indication. Nevertheless, through an intensive training of physicians in ICD-implantation, device replacement, programming, and aftercare of ICD patients, as well as the use of newer SVT discrimination and lead monitoring algorithms the rate of potential risks can be reduced substantially.

Author details

Damir Erkapic[1] and Tamas Bauernfeind[2]

1 University of Giessen and Marburg, Medical Clinic I, Department of Cardiology, Giessen, Germany and Kerckhoff Heart and Thorax Center, Department of Cardiology, Bad Nauheim, Germany

2 SRH Zentralklinikum Suhl gGmbH, Internal Medicine I, Department of Cardiologly, Suhl, Germany

References

[1] Wilkoff BL, Auricchio A, Brugada J, Cowie M, Ellebogen KA, Gillis AM, Hayes dL, Howlett JG, Kautzner J, Love CJ, Morgan JM, Priori SG, Reynolds DW, Schoenfeld MH, Vardas PE. HRS/EHRA Expert Consensus on the Monitoring of Cardiovascular Implantable Electronic Devices (CIEDs): description of techniques, indications, personnel, frequency and ethical considerations: developed in partnership with the Heart Rhythm Society (HRS) and the European Heart Rhythm Association (EHRA); and in collaboration with the American College of Cardiology (ACC), the American Heart Association (AHA), the European Society of Cardiology (ESC), the Heart Failure Association of ESC (HFA), and the Heart Failure Society of America (HFSA). Endorsed by the Heart Rhythm Society, the European Heart Rhythm Association (a registered branch of the ESC), the American College of Cardiology, the American Heart Association. Europace 2008;10:707-725.

[2] Tchou P, Axtell K, Anderson AJ, Keim S, Sra J, Trooup P, Jazayeri M, Avitall B, Akhtar M. When is it safe not to replace an implantable cardioverter defibrillator generator? Pacing ClinElectrophysiol 1991;14:1875-1880.

[3] Grimm W, Marchlinski FE. Shock occurrence in patients with an implantable cardioverter-defibrillator without spontaneous shocks before first generator replacement for battery depletion. Am J Cardiol 1994;73:969-970.

[4] Dürsch M, Pitschner HF, Schwarz T, Sperzel J, König S, Bahavar H, Klövekorn WP, Neuzner J. Therapy with implanted cardioverter-defibrillator: Is a replacement of the impulse generator due to battery depletion also necessary without the occurrence of a tachyarrhythmia episode? Z Kardiol 1998;87:32-37.

[5] Tandri H, Griffith LS, Tang Tm Nasir K, Zardkoohi O, Reddy CV, Capps M, Calkins H, Donahue JK. Clinical course and long-term follow-up of patients receiving implantable cardioverter-defibrillators. Heart Rhythm 2006;3:762-768.

[6] Koller MT, Schaer B, Wolbers M, Sticherling C, Bucher HC, Osswald S. Death without prior appropriate implantable cardioverter-defibrillator therapy. A competing risk study. Circulation 2008;117:1918-1926.

[7] Borleffs CJW, van Erven L, Schotman M, Boersma E, Kies P, Borger van der Burg AE, Zeppenfeld K, Bootsma M, van der Wall EE, Bax JJ, Schalij MJ. Recurrence of ventricular arrhytmias in ischaemic secondary prevention implantable cardioverter defibrillator recipients: long-term follow-up of the Leiden out-of-hospital cardiac arrest study (LOHCAT). Eur Heart J 2009;30:1621-1626.

[8] Erkapic D, Sperzel J, Stiller S, Meltendorf U, Mermi J, Wegscheider K, Hügl B for the INSURE investigators. Long term benefit of ICD therapy after elective device replacement: results of the incidence free survival after ICD replacement (INSURE) trial – a prospective multicenter study. Eur Heart J 2012, doi:10.1093/eurheartj/ehs177

[9] Alsheikh-Ali AA, Homer M, Maddukuri PV, Kalsmith B, Estes III NAM, Link MS. Time-Dependence of appropriate implantable defibrillator therapy in patients with ischemic cardiomyopathy. J CardiovascElectrophyiol. 2008;19:784-789.

[10] Goldenberg I, Gillespie J, Moss AJ, Hall WJ, Klein H, McNitt S, Brown MW, Cygankiewicz I, Zareba W, and the Executive Committee of the Multicenter Automatic Defibrillator Implantation Trial II. Long-Term Benefit of Primary Prevention With an Implantable Cardioverter-Defibrillator An Extended 8-Year Follow-Up Study of the Multicenter Automatic. Circulation 2010;122:1265-1271.

[11] Wilkoff BL, Cook JR, Epstein AE, Greene HL, Hallstrom AP, Hsia H, Kutalek SP, Sharma A; dual chamber and VVI implantable defibrillator trial investigators. Dual-chamber pacing or ventricular backup pacing in patients with an implantable defibrillator: the dual chamber and VVI implantable defibrillator (DAVID) trial. JAMA 2002;288:3115-3123.

[12] Van Welsenes GH, van Rees JB, Borleffs CJW, Cannegieter SC, Bax JJ, van Erven L, Schalij MJ. Long-term follow up of primary and secondary prevention implantable cardioverter defibrillator patients. Europace 2011;13:389-394.

[13] Van Welsenes GH, van Rees JB, Thijssen J, Trines SA, van ErvenLieselot, Schalij MJ, Borleffs CJW. Primary prevention implantable cardioverter Defibrillator recipients: the need for defibrillator back-up after an event-free first battery service-life. J CardiovascElectrophysiol 2011;22:1346-1350.

[14] Swygman C, Wang PJ, Link MS, Homoud MK, Estes III NA. Advances in implantable cardioverter defibrillators. CurrOpinCardiol 2002;17:24-28.

[15] Erkapic D, Amberger F, Bushoven P, Ehrlich J. More safety with more energy: survival of electrical storm with 40-J shocks. HerzschrittmachertherElektrophysiol 2011;22:252-254.

[16] Whellan DJ, Droogan CJ, Fitzpatrick J, Adams S, McCarey MM, Andrel J, Mather P, Rubin S, Bonita R, Keith S. Change in intrathoracic impedance measures during acute decompensated heart failure admission: results from the diagnostic data for discharge in heart failure patients (3D-HF) pilot study. J Card Fail 2012;18:107-112.

[17] Sarkar S, Hettrick DA, Koehler J, Rogers T, Grinberg Y, Yu CM, Abraham WT, Small R, Tang WH. Improved algorithm to detect fluid accumulation via intrathoracic impedance monitoring in heart failure patients with implantable devices. J Card Fail 2011;17:569-576.

[18] Brachmann J, Böhm M, Rybak K, Klein G, Butter C, Klemm H, Schomburg R, Siebemair J, Israel C, Sinha AM, Drexler H; OptiLink HF study executive board and Investigators. Fluid status monitoring with a wireless network to reduce cardiovascular-related hospitalizations and mortality in heart failure: rationale and design of the OptiLink Study (optimization of heart failure management using Optivol fluid status monitoring and Carelink). Eur J Heart Fail 2011;13:796-804.

[19] Papavasileiou LP, Forleo GB, Romeo F. Early detection of chronic myocardial ischemia in a patient implanted with an ICD capable of intracardiac electrogram monitoring. J invasive Cardiol 2011;23:532-533.

[20] Kleemann T, Becker T, Doenges K, Vater M, Senges J, Schneider S, Saggau W, Weisse U, Seidl K: Annual rate of transvenous defibrillation lead defects in implantable cardioverter-defibrillators over a period of > 10 years. Circulation 2007; 115:2474-2480.

[21] Kodoth V, Cromie N, Lau E, McEneaney D, Wilson C, Roberts, MJ. Riata lead failure: a report from Northern Ireland Riata lead screening programme. Eur Heart J 2011;32: Suppl, 310. (Abstract P1838).

[22] Erkapic D, Duray GZ, Bauernfeind T, De Rosa S, Hohnloser SH. Insulation defects of thin high-voltage ICD leads: an underestimated problem? J CardiolvascElectrophysiol 2011;22:1018-1022.

[23] Schmutz M, Delacrétaz E, Schwick N, Roten L, Fuhrer J, Boesch C, Tanner H. Prevalence of asymptomatic and electrically undetectable intracardiac inside-out abrasion in silicon-coated Riata and Riata ST implantable cardioverter-defibrillator leads.Int J Cardiol 2012 [Epub ahead of print].

[24] Parvathaneni SV, Ellis CR, Rottman JN. High prevalence of insulation failure with externalized cables in St. Jude Medical Riata family ICD leads: Fluoroscopic grading scale and correlation to extracted leads. Heart Rhythm 2012 [Epub ahead of print].

[25] Jenney C, Tan J, Karicherla A, Burke J, Helland J: A new insulation material for cardiac leads with potential for improved performance. Heart Rhythm 2005; 2:S318-S319.

[26] Hauser RG, Kallinen KM, Almquist AD, Gornick CC, Katsiyiannis WT. Early failure of a small-diameter high voltage implantable cardioverter-defibrillator lead. Heart Rhythm 2007;4:892-896.

[27] Birnie DH, Parkash R, Exner DV, Essebag V, Healey JS, Verma A, Coutu B, Kus T, Mangat I, Ayala-Paredes F, Nery P, Wells G, Krahn AD. Clinical predictors of Fidelis lead failure: report from the Canadian Heart Rhythm Society Device Committee. Circulation 2012;125:1217-1225.

[28] Gold MR, Ahmad S, Browne K, Berg KC, Thackeray L, Berger RD. Prospective comparison of discrimination algorithms to prevent inappropriate ICD therapy: primary results of the Rhythm ID Going Head to Head Trial. Heart Rhythm 2012;9:370-377.

[29] Powell BD, Asirvatham SJ, Perschbacher DL, Jones PW, Cha YM, Cesario DA, Cao M, Gilliam Iii FR, Saxon LA. Noise, Artifact, and Oversensing Related Inappropriate ICD Shock Evaluation: ALTITUDE NOISE Study. Pacing ClinElectrophysiol 2012 doi: 10.1111/j.1540-8159.2012.03407.x. [Epub ahead of print].

[30] Kleemann T, Hochadel M, Strauss M, Skarlos A, Seidl K, Zahn R. Comparison Between Atrial Fibrillation-Triggered Implantable Cardioverter-Defibrillator (ICD)

Shocks and Inappropriate Shocks Caused by Lead Failure: Different Impact on Prognosis in Clinical Practice. J CardiovascElectrophysiol 2012 doi: 10.1111/j.1540-8167.2011.02279.x. [Epub ahead of print].

[31] Jordan J, Sperzel J. Psychocardiological practice guidelines for ICD implantation and long-term care. HerzschrittmachertherElektrophysiol 2011 Sep;22:140-145.

[32] Poole JE. Shocks: the whole truth, the partial truth, or nowhere near the truth. CircArrhythmElectrophysiol 2011;4:424-425.

[33] Cao J, Gillberg JM, Swerdlow CD. A fully automatic, implantable cardioverter-defibrillator algorithm to prevent inappropriate detection of ventricular tachycardia or fibrillation due to T-wave oversensing in spontaneous rhythm. Heart Rhythm 2012; 9:522-530.

[34] Auricchio A, Meijer A, Kurita T, Schloss E, Brinkman K, Claessens-van Ooijen M, Sterns L. Safety, efficacy, and performance of new discrimination algorithms to reduce inappropriate and unnecessary shocks: the PainFree SST clinical study design.Europace 2011;13:1484-1493.

[35] Birnie DH, Parkash R, Exner DV, Essebag V, Healey JS, Verma A, Coutu B, Kus T, Mangat I, Ayala-Paredes F, Nery P, Wells G, Krahn AD. Clinical predictors of Fidelis lead failure: report from the Canadian Heart Rhythm Society Device Committee. Circulation 2012;125:1217-1225.

[36] Kallinen LM, Hauser RG, Tang C, Melby DP, Almquist AK, Katsiyiannis WT, Gornick CC. Lead integrity alert algorithm decreases inappropriate shocks in patients who have Sprint Fidelis pace-sense conductor fractures. Heart Rhythm 2010;7:1048-1055.

[37] Gelder RN, Gunderson BD. Prevention of inappropriate ICD shocks due to lead insulation failure by continuous monitoring and automatic alert. Pacing ClinElectrophysiol 2012;35:e150-153. doi: 10.1111/j.1540-8159.2011.03316.x. [Epub ahead of print].

[38] Krahn AD, Lee DS, Birnie D, Healey JS, Crystal E, Dorian P, Simpson CS, Khaykin Y, Cameron D, Janmohamed A, Yee R, Austin PC, Chen Z, Hardy J, Tu JV; Ontario ICD Database Investigators. Predictors of short-term complications after implantable cardioverter-defibrillator replacement: results from the Ontario ICD Database.CircArrhythmElectrophysiol 2011;4:136-142.

Chapter 6

ICD in the Era of Telecardiology

J. Taieb, J. Bouet, R. Morice, J. Hourdain, B. Jouve,
Y. Rahal, T. Benchaa, H. Khachab, O. Rica and
C. Barnay

Additional information is available at the end of the chapter

http://dx.doi.org/10.5772/53361

1. Introduction

Home monitoring of Pacemakers trans-telephonically was introduced in 1971 and remained until recently the main technology to remotely follow the performance of PMs. It was mostly aimed at ascertaining the integrity of the system especially with regard to battery performance and longevity, appropriate capture, and sensing.

Modern Remote wireless communication from the Cardiac implantable electronic devices (CIED) to a home communicator allows the transmission of the information gathered by the device regarding programming, test and alerts, to the clinician. It became the new standard for remote follow-up. [1-3]

The current CIEDs being interrogated remotely include implantable cardioverter defibrillator (ICDs), pacemakers, implantable loop recorders and implantable haemodynamic monitors. [2]

2. Definitions and principles of telecardiology applicable to ICDs

Telecardiology or home monitoring of ICDs refers to remote communication technology in general. Different types of data transmission are available.

2.1. Type of transmissions

Remote follow-up refers to programmable scheduled transmissions in which routine CIED parameters are collected remotely in a format similar to that obtained during a routine clinic visit. As opposed to trans-telephonically monitoring, practically all information available during traditional ICD interrogation with a programmer can be obtained via remote follow-up for a better outcome of patients [4-5]

Remote monitoring is an alert function. It refers to data acquired automatically with unscheduled transmissions of any pre-specified alerts related to device functioning or to clinical events. The latter adds a new functionality to implanted devices, opening a new era of potentially beneficial pre-emptive interventions that may alter the natural history of a particular disease or condition. [6-7].

Patient-initiated interrogations refers to non-scheduled follow-up interrogations as a result of a patient experiencing a real or perceived clinical event, for which the patient is seeking expert evaluation.

2.2. Technology of transmission

Unlike traditional follow up that implies a clinic appointment, transportation and face to face meeting, remote follow up is based on Data transmitted from the device to the home monitoring station by wireless communication or using a telemetry head (for older models) between device and home monitoring station. This home monitor is linked by telephone (*analogic line or GSM*) to a central server or website automatically to deposit encrypted data for further analysis (figure 1).

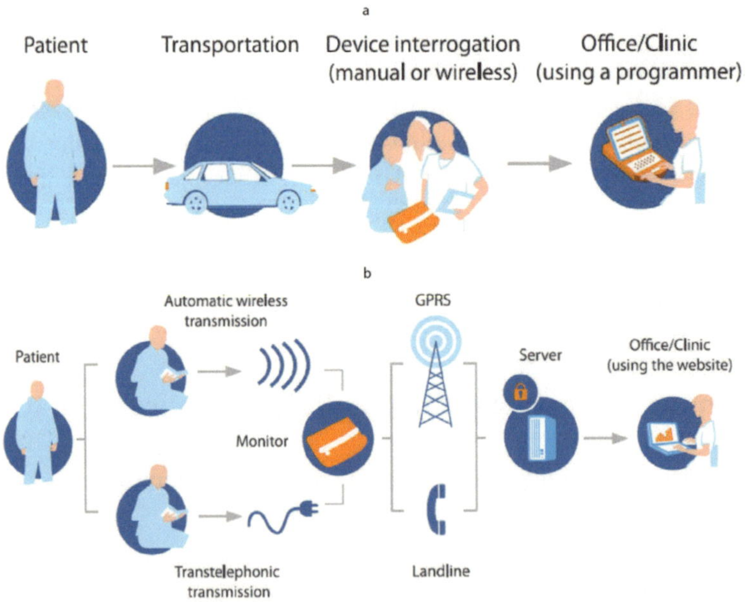

Figure 1. In clinic follow up (a) needs scheduling and transportation while Remote communication (b) is performed by a radiofrequency transmitter circuitry integrated in the ICD utilizing telephone lines or cellular phone technology. The ICD transfers encrypted data via the Transmitter to a service centre using a cellular network. The service centre provides a cardiologic report accessible online by the physician via a secure Internet access

http://dx.doi.org/10.5772/53361

Alert notifications are sent to physicians via pager, fax, SMS, voice message, or email. Many systems require access to a dedicated (device or company specific) website to obtain detailed information on the interrogation.

Remote reprogramming of alert level (yellow or red) is possible but remote ICD programming is not yet available in clinical practice, mainly due to safety considerations regarding data protection and unauthorized control of device function.

ICD compatible with home monitoring use radiofrequency telemetry to send information to a home communicator. This feature allows also the device to be operated remotely on a short distance (3 to 7 meters) during implantation procedure hence more flexibility, shorter intervention time, and lower risk of infection.[8] Radiofrequency telemetry is also very useful during in person follow up, eliminating the need for patient preparation and ECG monitoring in most cases, all information being accessible via the programmer (figure 2). Unfortunately, this possibility of short distance remote ICD interrogation and programming is not fully available for all brands at this time. (table 1)

	Boston Scientific Latitude	**Biotronik Home Monitoring**	**Medtronic CareLink**	**St Jude Merlin.net**	**Sorin SMARTVIEW**
Network	Analogue phone line.	GSM network (Europe & USA), Analogue phone line (USA &Japan) 3G (Japan)	Analogue phone line and GSM network	Analogue phone line, cellular network and WiFi	Analogue phone line and GSM network
Physician notification	Fax, phone, email	SMS, email, fax	SMS, email	Fax, email, SMS and automated phone calls	Fax, email, SMS
IEGM (real-time at remote follow-up)	10 s	30 s	10 s	30 s	7 s
FDA and CE Mark system approval	Yes	Yes	Yes	Yes	CE yes FDA (in progress)
Short distance RF remote programming	Yes	Yes (available in 2012)	Yes	Yes with an antenna	no

Table 1. Comparaison of communications features

a

b

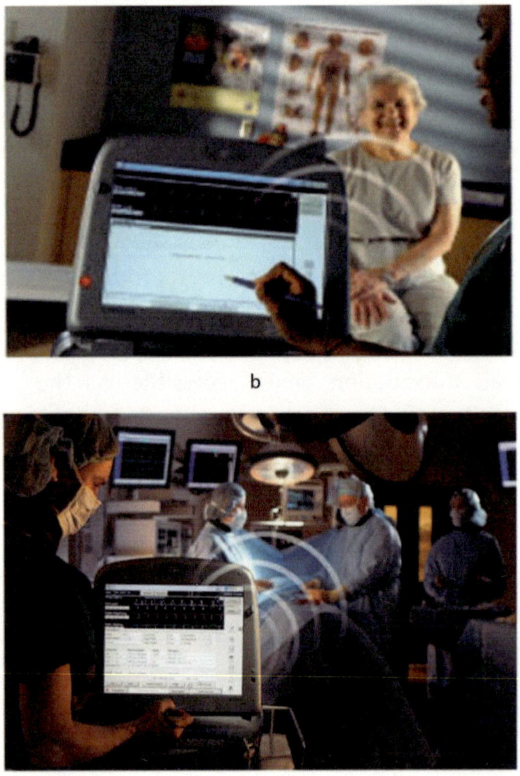

Figure 2. Some manufacturers use RF to interrogate and program remotely on a short distance. This is of particular interest during in person follow up (a) and during implantation procedure (b)

2.3. Types of alerts

The ability of implantable devices to continuously monitor variables such as heart rate, [9,10] the patient's daily activities, [11] intrathoracic impedance for the detection of fluid accumulation, [12] the occurrence of arrhythmias [13,14] and the integrity of the system [15] may provide early warning of changes in cardiac status or of safety issues and allow timely management. When these patients have clinical events such as ICD shocks or device audible alert notifications of possible critical situations, they often visit the emergency department or clinic for an unscheduled examination.

ICD and lead dysfunction may be associated with severe consequences and could be anticipated thanks to home monitoring alerts. Patients could be contacted to correct the problem in office for reprogramming or in hospital if a procedure is needed. [16-17]

Significant change in lead impedance, pacing or sensing thresholds, could be linked to lead failure and should be investigated thoroughly. It has been reported that remote monitoring helps prevent inappropriate shocks in a population at risk. [18]

http://dx.doi.org/10.5772/53361

An hemodynamic measurement modification, a low rate of resynchronisation should lead physicians to look for an aetiology (e.g. atrial fibrillation, Av delay, crosstalk…) in order to avoid a cardiac heart failure.

Development of persistent atrial fibrillation with fast ventricular rate close to ventricular fibrillation (VF) zone, frequent episodes of ventricular tachycardia (VT) with delivery of frequent antitachycardiac pacing sequences, should also act as a trigger for a follow up visit in order to change ICD parameters (VT, VF Zones, discrimination algorithms), or drug therapy.

2.4. Home monitor communicator

This is a remote telemetry device able to communicate with the ICD automatically in real time or at scheduled intervals, and that transmits the encrypted data over long distances utilizing telephone lines or cellular phone technology. The data are then entered and stored in dedicated servers that act as data repositories and communicate actively or passively with the caregivers of the patient. A specific home communicator was developed by each company: Medtronic Care- Link, Boston Scientific Latitude, Biotronik Home Monitoring, Sorin Smart View and St Jude Merlin@Home.net. In the near future, all systems will be compatible with GSM. Besides, Biotronik offers complete mobility of the home monitoring station with battery backup. Furthermore, frequency of remote follow up, and selection of remote monitoring alerts are fully programmable in all systems

3. Advantages and challenges of telecardiology

3.1. Physicians

Because of the burden of follow-up of ICD patients, with regular in-office visits every 3-6 months, puts on specialized electrophysiology clinics Heidbuchel et al. [19] retrospectively evaluated in 1739 ICD visits in a random set of 169 patients. The standard follow-up scheme consisted of in office visits 1 month after implantation and then every 6 months, unless approaching battery depletion. They conclude that ICD remote monitoring can potentially diagnose 99.5% of arrhythmia or device-related problems if combined with a follow-up by the local general practitioner and/or referring cardiologist. Its use may provide a way to significantly reduce in-office follow-up visits that are a burden for both hospitals and patients. A similar study was performed by Elsner et al. [20]. They investigated in a prospective, randomized, and multicentre comparison study the effect of ICD home monitoring against conventional follow-up in 115 MADIT II patients. The results prove that the simplified ICD follow-up scheme with additional home monitoring in MADIT II patients can reduce the number of visits and lead to time reduction.

In 2011 Boriani et al. published a survey [21] indicating that in 'real-world' clinical practice, the follow-up of CIEDs requires important resources in terms of time dedicated by specialized personnel, corresponding to cardiologists, nurses, internal technicians, and also, external, industry-employed technicians.

More recently Cronin et al. [22] found that analysis of remote monitoring transmissions has significant implications for device clinic workflow. Non-actionable transmissions are rapidly processed, allowing clinicians to focus on clinically important findings.

According to Theuns et al. [24]: "remote monitoring is feasible, may facilitate ICD follow up, and lead to early detection of system-related complications. Continuous monitoring of specific device parameters may avoid unnecessary replacements of devices or leads. However, as with every new technology, there are areas of uncertainty. Remote monitoring is associated with a redesigned organization of the care system, including physicians, allied professionals, and a dedicated remote monitoring service. Another area of uncertainty is related to the question of liability. The now "virtual patient" poses a paradigm shift. Physicians have the responsibility for responding to the new sources of data. How fast must a physician react to the transmitted alerts? Do we need 24 hours, 7 days a week coverage or is it legally acceptable not to check event notifications outside the office hours ? The development of practice guidelines on the appropriate role of remote monitoring of patients with implanted cardiac devices would help to address many of these issues."

3.2. Patients

Besides the decrease in number of in office follow up, safety and more rapid detection of actionable events compared with conventional monitoring in patients with implantable electronic cardiac devices were demonstrated in several studies:

In Lumos-T Safely Reduces Routine Office Device Follow-up (TRUST) multicentre trial [27, 28] authors concluded that home monitoring detected more device related issues and earlier compared with those following calendar-based or symptom-driven in-person interrogations. The results confirmed that conventional in-person follow-up methods underreport device malfunctions.

In the AWARE Study [29], Lazarus et al. analysed transmissions of 11624 recipients: 4631 pacemakers, 6548 single or dual chamber defibrillators and 445 cardiac resynchronisation therapy defibrillators (CRT-D) systems. The mean interval between the last follow-up and the occurrence of events notified by home monitoring was 26 days, representing a putative temporal gain of 154 and 64 days in patients usually followed up at 6 and 3 month intervals, respectively.

In 2010, the ALTITUDE registry showed that for the 69556 ICD and CRT-D patients receiving remote follow-up on the network, 1 and 5 year survival rates were higher compared with those in the 116 222 patients who received device follow-up in device clinics only (50% reduction; p=0.0001) [30].

Another example of remote monitoring improving clinical outcomes is its potential to reduce symptomatic lead failures, consisting of inappropriate shocks and symptomatic pacing inhibition due to oversensing. A study of patients who underwent repeat surgery due to malfunctions of the ICD lead compared the rate of symptomatic lead failure in patients monitored remotely with those followed up in-clinic [31]. Inappropriate shocks occurred in 27.3% of the remote group compared with 46.5% of the in-clinic group. This trend gains statistical significance if the compound endpoint of inappropriate shocks and symptomatic pacing inhibition due to oversensing is focused; 27.3% in the remote group compared with 53.4% in the in-clinic group. The remote monitoring system sent alert messages in 91% of all incidents, enabling intervention to prevent aninappropriate shock.

Mabo reported in the EVATEL study [32], a randomized trial that included 1500 patients implanted with single or dual chamber ICD that "Home monitoring leads to a decrease of 37% of inappropriate shocks.

Kacet reported similar results in the ECOST study [33]: "home monitoring reduces by 76% the number of aborted ICD charges with a significant impact on battery status and device longevity".

Raatikainen et al. [34] reported that over 90% of patients found the system easy to use. Marzegalli et al. [35] also reported that the review procedure was successful. Its mean duration was 5 ±2 minutes per transmission and users indicated that both access and navigation were easy. Patients reported a general preference for remote versus in clinic follow-up and described a sense of reassurance created by the remote monitoring capacity. In a study of 379 patients implanted with pacemakers, Halimi et al. reported all differences in the SF-36 questionnaire scores to be non-statistically significant [36]. Patient satisfaction was studied recently by Petersen et al. [23]: of the 385 of the patients that answered the survey (81.2%), ninety-five percent were content with the remote Follow up. Only 25% had unscheduled transmissions and most unscheduled transmissions were for appropriate reasons. Eighty-four percent of the patients wished for a more detailed response and 21% wished for a faster reply after routine transmissions.

Current ICDs provide not only arrhythmia information but also several indicators of heart failure (HF). Studies are under way to evaluate the benefits of HF specifics diagnostics coupled with home monitoring [25, 26].

3.3. Health economics

While remote monitoring (RM) may be able to reduce the time spent on device follow up it is not clear whether this relates to an overall reduction in costs. RM has its own costs including the cost of the transmitter, the setup and maintenance of the central server and database, patient and clinic staff education and staff time to read, interpret, import information into electronic medical records and act on transmission events/problems. The frequency of in office visits and the frequency of RM transmissions, proximity of the patient to the clinic and many other factors will affect the economic modeling as to the potential cost savings associated with RM. Beyond assessing the simple economic modeling is the assessment of cost effectiveness which also needs to consider the improvement in patient outcomes as well as the costs involved for each form of follow up.

3.4. Limits of telecardiology

A network failure may delay transfer of data. Most of telecardiology departments do not have 24/7services. Thus, an alert message issued on a Friday night has a good chance not to be examined before the following Monday. In addition transferred data through the network are privileged, leading to legal considerations regarding reliability of the technology and confidentiality especially during emergency situations. To add another level of complexity, each country seems to have a different modus operandi at this point in time.

Health care providers and health care organizations that are involved in remote monitoring (RM) of ICDs will typically sign a 'Terms of Use' agreement with each of the ICD vendors. These legal documents outline the provisions of RM between the ICD vendor and the user. The patient needs to be informed of the purpose and limitations of RM, such as the fact that it does not replace an emergency service or absence of dealing with alert events outside office hours. Before initiating RM and follow-up, the patient may be requested to sign a written informed consent stating these points and authorizing transmission of personal data to third parties, respect of privacy, and confidentiality of patient data by device companies should be subjected to strict rules, described in contracts. Cardiac implantable devices record a wealth of information and as devices become more sophisticated the scope of information can be expected to grow. Guidelines need to be established to determine the periodicity with which ICD transmissions would need to be reviewed and documented.

Vulnerability of security breaches by hackers accessing devices with wireless capability must be tested in every system. There have been no reports to date of unauthorized reprogramming of implantable devices; however, unauthorized access to personal information stored on internet servers must be also considered.

In addition, transfer of ICD data would be impossible if the home monitoring station is not close to the patient at reasonable time intervals. This could be happening in case of hospitalization in another center. The patient could even experience serious system failure without any data transmission.

Logistics may also be a limit to the development of home monitoring: It is up to the implanting center to organize ordering, stock management and traceability of home monitoring stations as well as patient education. The Sorin group is the only one so far using a distribution network to handle all these tasks.

3.5. Reimbursement

Reimbursement is important to the manufacturer in order to compensate for some of the costs related to the home monitoring stations and the transmission network. It remains a major concern in most countries, limiting the increase of use of remote monitoring despite growing evidence in favor of this technology. Today's cost containment pressure requires increased reimbursement efforts with the burden of proof shifting to medical communities and manufacturers. Reimbursement assessments often begin with the presumption that a technology or service will not be covered unless its use is supported by scientific evidence of improved outcomes. Recent publications like the EVOLVO study [37] are important milestones in this endeavor. It concludes that "remote monitoring can reduce emergency department/urgent in office visits and, in general, total healthcare use in heart failure patients with modern ICD/ CRT-D. Compared with standard follow-up through in-office visits and audible ICD alerts, remote monitoring results in increased efficiency for healthcare providers and improved quality of care for patients". Another study is under way to develop a cost minimization analysis from the hospital perspective and a cost effectiveness analysis from the third payer standpoint, based on direct estimates of costs and QOL associated with remote follow-ups, compared with standard ambulatory follow-ups, in the management of ICD and CRT-D recipients [38].

4. Conclusion

Remote monitoring of ICDs represents a growing area with increasing numbers of patients being subject to these technologies but also more and more physicians involved in decision making on the indications for these technologies and the handling of data in the context of clinical decision making.

Cardiac implantable device transmissions may occur either over telephone lines or over cellular network lines. These transmissions often only take less than a minute to a few minutes to complete. However, in the foreseeable future we can expect alternative methods of data transmission to become available with transmission rates that will make it possible for nearly continuous and instantaneous patient ICD data delivered to health care providers. There are, of course, limitations to how frequently ICD data can be reviewed by health care providers and battery longevity constraints will likely limit the transmission times as well.

Technological advancements continue to structure our practice of medicine, but with it often new legal challenges emerge. In order to minimize risk to patient and liability to health care providers a clear discussion regarding the expectations and limitations of remote monitoring between patients and health care providers is recommended

Acknowledgements

The authors thank Muriel Bon, Michelle Hartenstein, Xavier Laroche, Ariane Szczygiel, Marion De Matteis, Moti Daswani and Vincent Desplat for their expert technical assistance, and Fabrice Chomienne, for his help in the composition of the manuscript.

Author details

J. Taieb, J. Bouet, R. Morice, J. Hourdain, B. Jouve, Y. Rahal, T. Benchaa, H. Khachab, O. Rica and C. Barnay

Hospital Center of Aix en Provence, France

References

[1] Wilkoff BL, Auricchio A, Brugada J et al. HRS/
EHRA expert consensus on the monitoring of Cardiovascular Implantable Electronic Devices (CIEDs). Europace 2008;10:707-25.

[2] Dubner S, Auricchio A, Steinberg JS, et al SHNE/EHRA expert consensus on remote monitoring of cardiovascular implantable electronic devices (CIEDs) Annals of Non-invasive Electrocardiology 2012;17:35-36

[3] Winters SL, Packer DL, Marchlinski FE et al. North American Society of Electrophysiology and Pacing. Consensus statement on indications, guidelines for use, and recommendations for follow-up of implantable cardioverter-defibrillators. Pacing Clin Electrophysiol 2001;24:262 – 9.

[4] Crossley GH, Chen J, Choucair W, et al, on behalf of the PREFER Study Investigators. Clinical benefits of remote versus transtelephonic monitoring of implanted pacemakers. J Am Coll Cardiol 2009;54:2012–9.

[5] Crossley G, Boyle A, Vitense H, et al. The Clinical Evaluation of Remote Notification to Reduce Time to Clinical Decision (CONNECT) Trial. Am Heart J 2008;156:840–6

[6] Joseph GK, Wilkoff BL, Dresing T, et al. Remote interrogation and monitoring of implantable cardioverter defibrillators. J Interv Card Electrophysiol 2004;11:161 – 6

[7] Ricci RP, Morichelli L, Santini M. Home monitoring remote control of pacemaker and ICD patients in clinical practice. Impact on medical management and health care resource utilization. Europace 2008;10:164–70.

[8] Schoenfeld MH, Reynolds DW. Sophisticated remote implantable cardioverter defibrillator follow-up: a status report. Pacing Clin Electrophysiol 2005;28:235–40.

[9] Adamson PB, Smith AL, Abraham WT, et al; InSync III Model 8042 and Attain OTW Lead Model 4193 Clinical Trial Investigators. Continuous autonomic assessment in patients with symptomatic heart failure: prognostic value of heart rate variability measured by an implanted cardiac resynchronization device. Circulation. 2004;110:2389 –2394.

[10] Landolina M, Gasparini M, Lunati M, et al; InSync/InSync ICD Italian Registry Investigators. Heart rate variability monitored by the implanted device predicts response to CRT and long-term clinical outcome in patients with advanced heart failure. Eur J Heart Fail. 2008;10:1073–1079.

[11] Kadhiresan VA, Pastore J, Auricchio A et al; PATH-CHF Study Group. Pacing therapies in congestive heart failure: a novel method—the activity log index—for monitoring physical activity of patients with heart failure. Am J Cardiol. 2002;89: 1435–1437.

[12] Yu CM, Wang L, Chau E, et al. Intrathoracic impedance monitoring in patients with heart failure: correlation with fluid status and feasibility of early warning preceding hospitalization. Circulation. 2005;112:841– 848.

[13] Capucci A, Santini M, Padeletti L, Gulizia M et al; Italian AT500 Registry Investigators. Monitored atrial fibrillation duration predicts arterial embolic events in patients suffering from bradycardia and atrial fibrillation implanted with antitachycardia pacemakers. J Am Coll Cardiol. 2005;46:1913–1920.

[14] Santini M, Gasparini M, Landolina M, et al cardiological centers participating in Clinica lService Project. Device detected atrial tachyarrhythmias predict adverse outcome in real-world patients with implantable biventricular defibrillators. J Am Coll Cardiol. 2011;57:167–172.

[15] Gunderson BD, Patel AS, Bounds CA, et al. An algorithm to predict implantable cardioverter defibrillator lead failure. J Am Coll Cardiol. 2004;44:1898 –1902

[16] Joseph GK, Wilkoff BL, Dresing T, et al. Remote interrogation and monitoring of implantable cardioverter defibrillators. J Interv Card Electrophysiol 2004;11:161–6.

[17] Ricci RP, Morichelli L, Santini M. Home monitoring remote control of pacemaker and ICD patients in clinical practice. Impact on medical management and healthcare resource utilization. Europace 2008;10:164–70.

[18] Banck Z,, Axtell K, , Brodhagen K, et al. Inappropriate Shocks in Patients With Fidelis® Lead Fractures: Impact of Remote Monitoring and the Lead Integrity Algorithm Journal of Cardiovasc Electrophysiol, 2011;22, :1107-1114,

[19] Heidbuchel H, Lioen P, Foulon S et al. Potential role of remote monitoring for scheduled and unscheduled evaluations patients with an implantable defibrillator. Europace 2008;10:351–7.

[20] Elsner C, Sommer P, Piorkowski C, et al. A Prospective Multicenter Comparison Trial of home monitoring against regular follow-up in MADIT II. Comput Cardiol 2006;33:241–4.

[21] Boriani G , Auricchio A, Klersy C, et al. Healthcare personnel resource burden related to in-clinic follow-up of cardiovascular implantable electronic devices: a European Heart Rhythm Association and Eucomed joint survey. Europace 2011 ;13 :1166–1173

[22] Cronin, E.M., Ching, E.A., Varma, N. et al, Remote monitoring of cardiovascular devices - a time and activity analysis, Heart Rhythm 2012, doi: 10.1016/j.hrthm. 2012.08.002.

[23] Helen H Petersen , Mie C Jensen Larsen, Olav W Nielsen, et al. Patient satisfaction and suggestions for improvement of remote ICD monitoring. J Interv Card Electrophysiol 2012 34:317–324

[24] Theuns D. A. M. J. ,Jordaens L. Use of remote monitoring in the management of system-related complications in implantable defibrillator patients. Neth Heart J 2012 20:82–85

[25] Brachmann J, l Bohm M, Rybak K, et al on behalf of the OptiLink HF Study Executive Board and Investigators. Fluid status monitoring with a wireless network to reduce cardiovascular-related hospitalizations and mortality in heart failure: rationale and design of the OptiLink HF Study (Optimization of Heart Failure Management using OptiVol Fluid Status Monitoring and CareLink). European Journal of Heart Failure 2011;13:796–804

[26] Sack S, Wende CM, Nagel H et al . Potential value of automated daily screening of cardiac resynchronization therapy defibrillator diagnostics for prediction of major cardiovascular events: results from Home-CARE (Home Monitoring in Cardiac Resynchronization Therapy) study European Journal of Heart Failure 2011;13:1019–1027

[27] Varma N, Michalski J, Epstein AE, et al. Automatic remote monitoring of ICD lead and generator performance: the TRUST trial. Circ Arrhythm Electrophysiol 2010;3:428–36.

[28] Varma N, Epstein A, Irimpen A, et al. The lumos-T safely reduces routine efficacy and safety of automatic remote monitoring for implantable cardioverter-defibrillator follow-up. The Lumos-T Safely Reduces Routine Office Device Follow-Up (TRUST) Trial. Circulation 2010;122:325–32.

[29] Lazarus A. Remote, wireless, ambulatory monitoring of implantable pacemakers, cardioverter defibrillators, and cardiac resynchronization therapy systems: analysis of a worldwide database. Pacing ClinElectrophysiol 2007;30(Suppl 1):S2–12.

[30] Saxon LA, Hayes DL, Gilliam FR et al. Long-term outcome after ICD and CRT implantation and influence of remote device follow-up: the ALTITUDE survival study. Circulation 2010;122:2359–67. Epub 2010 Nov 22.

[31] Spencker S, Coban N, Koch L, et al. A Potential role of home monitoring to reduce inappropriate shocks in implantable cardioverter defibrillator patients due to lead failure. Europace 2009;11:483–8.

[32] Mabo P. Remote follow-up of patients implanted with an ICD. The prospective randomized EVATEL study. European Society of Cardiology 2011. Hotline 2. 29 août 2011.

[33] Kacet S. Safety of implantable cardioverter defibrillator follow-up using remote monitoring : a randomized controlled trial. Session Hot Line 2. Congrès de l'European Society of Cardiology, Paris, 29 août 2011

[34] Raatikainen MJP et al. Remote monitoring of implantable cardioverter defibrillator patients: a safe, time-saving, and cost-effective means for follow-up Europace 2008;10(10):1145–51

[35] Marzegalli M et al. Remote Monitoring of CRT-ICD: The Multicenter Italian Care-Link Evaluation—Ease of Use, Acceptance, and Organizational Implications PACE 2008;31:1259–64

[36] Halimi F, Clementy J, Attuel P, et al, on behalf of the OEDIPE trial Investigators. Optimized post-operative surveillance of permanent pacemakers by home monitoring: the OEDIPE trial. Europace 2008;10:1392–9.

[37] Landolina M, ; Perego GB , Lunati M,et al. Remote Monitoring Reduces Healthcare Use andImproves Quality of Care in Heart Failure Patients WithImplantable DefibrillatorsThe Evolution of Management Strategies of Heart Failure Patients With Implantable Defibrillators (EVOLVO) Study. Circulation. 2012;125:2985-2992

[38] Ricci RP , D'Onofrio A, Padeletti L, et al. Rationale and design of the health economics evaluation registry for remote follow-up: TARIFF. Europace doi:10.1093/europace/eus093 in press

Section 4

ICD Implantation Procedure

Chapter 7

ICD and PM Implantation Procedure: Relevant Periprocedural Issues

Joern Schmitt

Additional information is available at the end of the chapter

http://dx.doi.org/10.5772/54203

1. Introduction

1.1. Perioperative management of antiplatelet and anticoagulation therapy

Over the last years implanting physicians are frequently forced to manage perioperative situation with increased bleeding risk due to anticoagulation (oral or intravenous) or dual antiplatelet therapy. Large number of patients have indication for long term use of oral anticoagulation because of atrial fibrillation, prosthetic heart valves, anamnestic cerebrovascular accident or recurrent venous thromboembolism. On the other hand an increasing number of patients have indication for dual antiplatelet therapy (DAPT) - mainly after coronary artery interventions. There is an increased need for a standardized perioperative management by either postponing the procedure (if clinically possible), bridging or pausing the therapy or taking the risk of a bleeding complication if inevitable. To help the implanting physician with a reasonable decision, there are guidelines offered by the large cardiology societies [1-4] concerning the management of patients with AF, as well as recent publications dealing with this increasing challenge [5-7].

1.2. Antiplatelet therapy

Antiplatelet therapy is usually indicated after coronary artery interventions, myocardial infarction as well as extracardial indications including cerebral infarction or peripheral artery disease. Following coronary intervention the need for dual antiplatelet therapy usually is temporally, the duration of therapy depending on the type of stent (bare metal Stent /BMS/ vs. drug eluting stent /DES/) as well as on the stent position and implant indication (acute coronary syndrome vs. elective angioplasty). Following this time period most patients will be put on aspirin therapy lifelong. Shortening the initially recommended time period of DAPT is highly discouraged due to high risk of stent thrombosis. On the other hand most PM and numerous ICD implants should not be postponed because of a potential or evident risk of syncope, asystoly or sudden cardiac death.

A review of recent studies shows interesting and relevant results concerning device implantations under DAPT. Patients underwent device implantation under DAPT (ASA and clopidogrel) suffered the highest rate of pocket hematomas and bleeding complications when compared to patients with ASA alone or oral anticoagulation. The risk of pocket hematoma in patients implanted under DAPT may as high as 20% in a smaller study (200 patients 10% with DAPT) [6]. Tompkins et al. retrospectively analyzed 1388 device implantations including 139 patients with DAPT, they found a 4-fold increased risk of bleeding complications compared to controls (7.2% vs. 1.6%) [7]. In this study patients receiving only ASA therapy had a bleeding risk more than 2-fold (3.9% vs. 1.6%) showing a trend to significance ($p=0.078$). Kutinsky et al. collected prospectively the data of 935 PM and ICD implantations concerning pocket hematomas. They described an overall bleeding risk of 9.5%, which was significantly increased in those on clopidogrel therapy (18.3%) [8]. Data concerning the "new" antiplatelet agents ticagrelor and prasugrel in device implantations are missing. Prasugrel showed to have a higher bleeding risk in the interventional and CABG parts of the TRITON-TIMI38 trial [9-11]. To which extend this may be extrapolated to device implantation is questionable. Ticagrelor showed a comparable bleeding risk to clopidogrel in the PLATO Trial [12, 13]. Again there is no explicit data on the risk of bleeding and hematoma in pacemaker or ICD implant procedures.

1.3. Oral anticoagulants

Besides antiplatelet therapy as concomitant treatment in cardiovascular patients there are many treated with oral anticoagulants (OAC) / vitamin K antagonists (VKA) needing a device implantation or revision. In the last years new drugs evolved in this field of anticoagulation with broad indication spectrum reaching from deep venous thrombosis prophylaxis and therapy up to the prevention of cardio-embolic events in atrial fibrillation. In contrast to the described dual antiplatelet therapy oral anticoagulation therapy for example in AF and after mechanical heart valve replacement is a lifelong therapy with a constant risk of thromboembolic and bleeding events. Thus postponing implantation procedure - even if clinically possible - is of little help. Three options arise when dealing with patients on oral anticoagulation: 1. Pausing OAC and bridging with unfractionated (UFH) or low molecular weight (LMWH) heparin, 2. Continue OAC and perform the implantation at a moderate INR (e.g. 1.5-2.0) if possible, 3. Pausing completely and reinitiating 3-5 days post implantation. In patients with the need for anticoagulation therapy the risk of thromboembolic events may be categorized into low, moderate or high by adopting and expanding the CHA_2DS_2-VASc-Score (table 1). The action taken should be adopted to this risk (table 2) [14].

http://dx.doi.org/10.5772/54203

Risk factor	Score
Congestive heart failure/LV-dysfunction	1
Hypertension	1
Age 65-74 years	1
Age ≥ 75 years	2
Diabetes mellitus	1
Stroke/TIA/thrombo-embolism	2
Vascular disease	1
Sex (female)	1
Total Maximum	9

Table 1. The CHA_2DS_2-VASc-Score

Score	Risk
0	0
1	1.3
2	2.2
3	3.2
4	4.0
5	6.7
6	9.8
7	9.6
8	6.7
9	15.2

Table 2. Adjusted stroke rate according to the CHA_2DS_2-VASc-Score

There are several publications dealing with device implantation in anticoagulated patients. Most of them evaluate the use/benefit of perioperative bridging therapy. Giudici et al reported a series of 1025 implants including 470 oral anticoagulated patients with a mean INR of 2.6 (±1). The rate of pocket hematoma was not significantly different between the two groups (OAC 2.6%, Controls 2.2%) [15]. Wiegand et al. reported their analysis of predictors of pocket hematoma in 3164 PM/ICD implants and generator exchanges [16]. Besides a described risk of hematoma formation of 3.1% under ASA and 21.7% under DAPT, a higher risk of hematoma formation could be found in patients were OAC therapy was bridged with

UFH perioperative. In this study two postoperative regiments were compared. One with a bolus of heparin immediate at the end of the procedure (2.500 IU to 5000 IU) followed by continuous infusion (target aPTT from 40-60s). The other group was started on continuous heparin infusion without a bolus within 12h post implantation with the same target aPTT. The risk of pocket hematoma was 28.1% in the bolus and 12% in the standard group. One further study reports data of a "head to head" comparison in CRT-implants between patients on OAC having an INR 2-3 perioperative, a second group having heparin bridging therapy and a third – control – group including patients where OAC was simply stopped for 4 days. It showed again that the incidence of pocket hematomas were significantly increased in patients where heparin bridging was performed: 20.7% vs. 5.0% in the OAC group and 4.1% in controls ($p=0.03$). Hematomas were responsible for longer in hospital stays (controls: 1.6 ± 1.6; warfarin group: 2.9 ± 2.7; bridging 3.7 ± 3.2; $p < 0.001$) [17].

It should be noted that the data of all the reported studies showed different rates of hematoma formation with and without anticoagulation or bridging therapy but no significantly different rate in the occurrence of thromboembolic events were described.

Furthermore, new anticoagulant agents became available recently: the oral direct thrombininhibitor dabigatran and the oral Factor Xa inhibitor rivaroxaban, both approved to prevent thromboembolic events in patients with non valvular atrial fibrillation as well as to prevent post surgery venous thrombosis. There are only limited data on bleeding complications in pacemaker and defibrillator implantation under therapy with one of these two new approved drugs. Data from the RELY trial (dabigatran) in patients (4591 patients) with AF and the need for an interventional procedure, including pacemaker/defibrillator implantation (10.3%) showed no significantly different risks for major bleeding when compared with warfarin (dabigatran 110 mg 3.8% or dabigatran 150 mg 5.1% or warfarin 4.6%) [18]. The median dabigatran discontinuation was 49 hours (25-85) ahead of the procedure compared to 114 hours (87-144) in patients on OAC. One study was evaluating the risk of major bleeding events after total hip or total knee arthroplasty in patients concomitantly treated with NSAIDS or ASA and dabigatran (2x110mg or 1x150mg daily) [19]. In this study no difference in major bleeding events could be observed, neither between dabigatran and enoxaparin treated patients nor between concomitantly treated patients.

A recent metaanalysis by Bernard et al. [20] showed an overall incidence of bleeding complications of 4.6% ranging from 2.2% in patients without any anticoagulation/antiplatelet therapy up to 14.6% in patients receiving a heparin bridging strategy. Calculated odds ratios compared to the no therapy group was 8.3 (95% CI 5.5-12.9) for heparin bridging strategy, 5.0 (95% CI 3.0-8.3) for dual antiplatelet therapy and 1.6 (95% CI 0.9-2.6) with continued oral anticoagulation. This again contributes to the idea that bridging therapy (despite high risk patients) is maybe not the best way to go.

1.4. Conclusion / recommendation

In our institution considering the above mentioned we decided to adopt a recommendation from Korantzopoulos et al. modified algorithm [21]. In patients undergoing generator replacement or Loop-Recorder implantation we continue the actual therapy, antiplatelet as

http://dx.doi.org/10.5772/54203

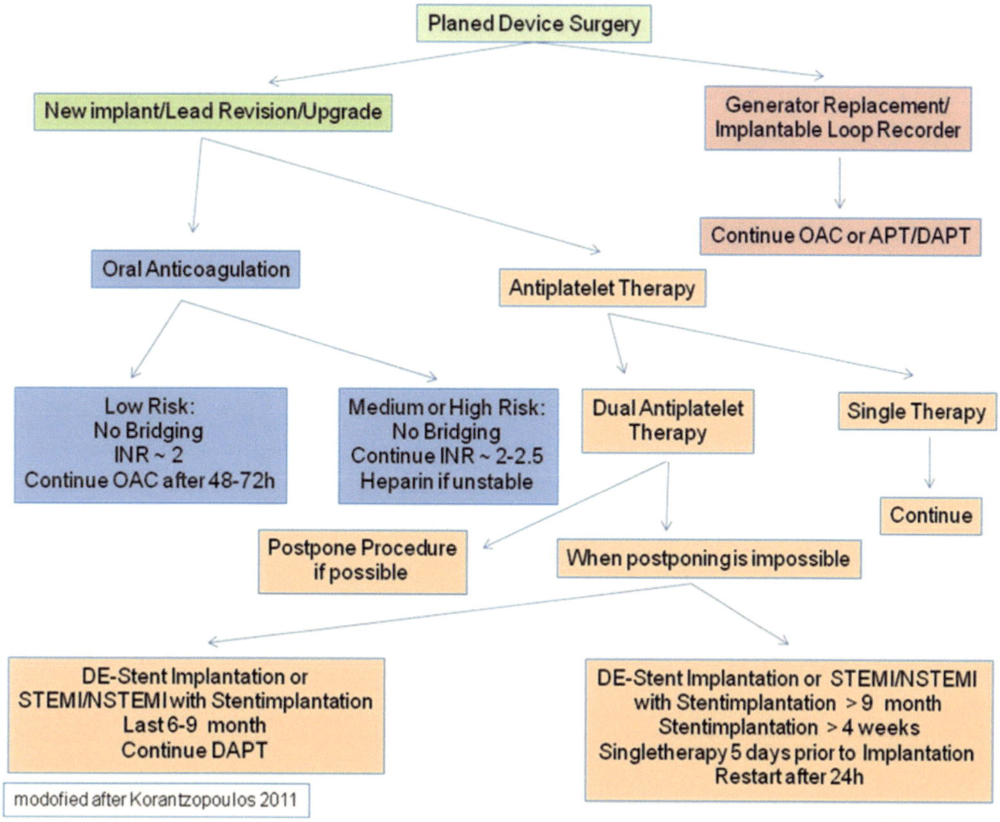

Scheme 1.

well as anticoagulation, aiming to an INR of max. 2.5. All new implantations, revisions or upgrades needing vascular access are managed differently – according to our flow chart (Scheme 1 - adopted and modified after Hofmeister and Korantzopoulos [14, 21]). If dual antiplatelet therapy is present we try to postpone the procedure, according to current guidelines depending on the indication for DAPT. The time with the need for DAPT depends on the used Stent(s) as well as the anatomic position and the indication itself (ACS vs. elective). In general DAPT is mandatory for at least 6 month, in patients after ACS as well as in patients with a drug eluting stent (DES). After non DES implantation DAPT has to be administered for at least 4 weeks. If postponing is impossible the implant-procedure would be performed under dual antiplatelet therapy and wide precautions. Single antiplatelet therapy would be continued.

In patients under oral anticoagulation therapy we apply table 1, 2 and 3 to estimate the patient´s risk for thromboembolic events. Patients with low risk will be operated with a break of OAC and an INR of up to 2.0. OAC will be resumed after 48h with the maintenance dose. Patients with medium risk will be operated with continued OAC and an INR of 2.0 2.5. High risk patients according to table 3 will be discussed and depending on the procedure either be operated with an INR close to 2.5 or heparin bridging therapy. We do not perform bridging with any type of heparin as a routine protocol. Oral Anticoagulation should be stopped approximately 3-5 days before the procedure, depending on the used substance as well the individual maintenance dose. Local haemostiptics or drainage will be used by the judgment of the operator.

Thromboembolic risk assessment in patients on oral anticoagulation		
Low thromboembolic risk (<5%/year)	Medium thromboembolic risk (5-10%/year)	High thromboembolic risk (>10%/year)
AF patients with CHA_2DS_2-VASc-Score 0-2 (but no TIA/CVA) Mechanical aortic valves (> 3 months) Post venous thromboembolism (>12 month)	AF patients with CHA_2DS_2-VASc-Score 3-5 Mechanical aortic valves + AF Malignancy ass. venous thromboembolism Multiple or current thromboembolism Valve repair/-exchange (<3months)	AF patients with CHA_2DS_2-VASc-Score 5-6 (or TIA/CVA <3months) Mechanical mitral valves Mechanical aortic valves + AF (CHA_2DS_2-VASc ≥2) Mechanical aortic valves (older models) Known thrombophilic disorder LV-thrombus

Table 3. Relative Risk assessment of perioperative thromboembolic events without anticoagulation therapy. Modified after Douketis JD, et al (2008) The perioperative management of antithrombotic therapy (ACCP Evidence-based clinical practice guidelines, 8th Edition). Chest 133:299–339 and De Caterina R, Husted S, Wallentin L et al (2007) Anticoagulants in heart disease: current status and perspectives. Eur Heart J 28:880–913

2. Perioperative antibiotic therapy

2.1. Introduction

Since the beginning of cardiac implantable electronic devices (CIED) prevention of device infection is a serious issue and is under permanent discussion [22-24].

Despite "optimal implantation procedure" concerning optimal sterility and hygienic conditions in terms of materials, implant room and process, there are several factors that pose a higher risk for CIED infections: device/pocket revision, use of temporary pacing leads before placement of the permanent device, central venous catheters, longer operative time and operator inexperience, development of postoperative pocket hematoma, diabetes mellitus, long-term use of corticosteroids and other immunosuppressive drugs and seperated focus of primary infection [25]. The use of perioperative antibiotics or the therapy of choice, as well as necessity and effect of flushing the wound with antiinfective detergents is under debate [26, 27]. There are newly developed antimicrobial device coatings which are not yet available [28, 29].

Described rates of implant related device infections in published studies have a wide range reaching from 0.13% to 19.9% with 0.5% of the patients developing endocarditis or sepsis as

http://dx.doi.org/10.5772/54203

a major complication [24, 30]. In addition to the severe or even lethal complication there is also an impact on health economics with estimated costs of up to 50.000$ per case [31, 32].

The daily routine of perioperative antibiotic administration to prevent infections of CIED is highly variable in terms of agents and dosage. It is generally accepted that a reduction of device infections can be achieved by this approach [33]. Regiments based on vancomycin, imipenem or cephazolin administered either perioperative as single shot or up to 3 days are known. In terms of evidence based medicine there are just 7 trials dealing with perioperative antibiotics in CIEDS up to 2009 [27, 30, 34]. They were consisted of small number of patients with very variable designs in terms of follow up duration, inclusion criteria, used antibiotic agent and definition of events. Thus varying results were reported and a definite conclusion could hardly be found. Four of those trials described a benefit in terms of reduction of device/system infections. Three did not describe any difference, however, in one study there was no infection at all in the included 106 patients [35]. Those trials were mainly conducted in the 1980´s – another limitation since implanted systems (generators and leads) as well as implant techniques underwent marked developments in the last 3 decades.

The most recent and relevant study was a double-blinded randomized trial by Oliveira et al. in 2009 [36]. In this study 649 consecutive ICD and pacemaker patients (first implant and generator replacement) were included and followed (fixed schedule for 6 month and additionally when clinically indicated). Randomization was made to either 1g of cephazolin or placebo directly prior operation. Allergic patients were excluded. The primary endpoint was the occurrence of infection, classified being one of the following: superficial, pocket or systemic infection. The two groups were balanced and no differences concerning the known risk factors for CIED infections were present. The study was interrupted after 26.5 month by the safety committee because of significant differences in the primary endpoint. CIED related infections occurred in 0.64% in the cephazolin group and 3.28% in the placebo group (p=0.016). The 13 patients that developed infections showed the typically germs all from the Staphylococcus-family. The time until infection after implantation was 11-33 days without a difference between the cephazolin and the placebo group. The multivariate analysis identified pocket hematoma and lack of antibiotic prophylaxis as independent risk factors for any kind of infection. Odds ratios were not calculated.

Based on the results of this study as well as previously published non randomized data antibiotic prophylaxis should be performed in any device related operation (implantation as well as generator replacement). In our institution cephazolin is administered - being the only evidence based antibiotic drug until now. In case of known allergy against cephazolin a single shot of 1g vancomycin seems the most appropriate alternative as most common species in CIED infection are staphylococci or streptococci [37, 38]. If the implanting hospital has a high prevalence of methicilin-resistant staphylococci (MRSA) vancomycin should be considered to be the first choice [33]. Some authors argue that in some regions with a very high prevalence of MRSA vancomycin should be even generally the first choice, however, this is not evidence based and should be considered carefully together with the local infectologist [33].

An interesting, newly developed approach of device coatings seems to be able to control local bacterial growth and thus is supposed to be able to prevent system infections [28, 29]. The study by Matl et al. describes the use of gentamycin and teicoplanin in a lipid-based drug delivery-system which was able to deliver high local concentrations over 96h and inhibit completely the growth of S. aureaus in vivo [28]. Wong et al. published data on a dual layer device coating, consisting of gentamycin to control local colonization/infection and diclofenac to control local inflammation due to tissue injury on top of a microbicidal base film [29]. In vitro they could show excellent results in terms of S. aureus control (figure 1). No data on extended in vivo use of any coating is yet available but the idea and techniques are promising.

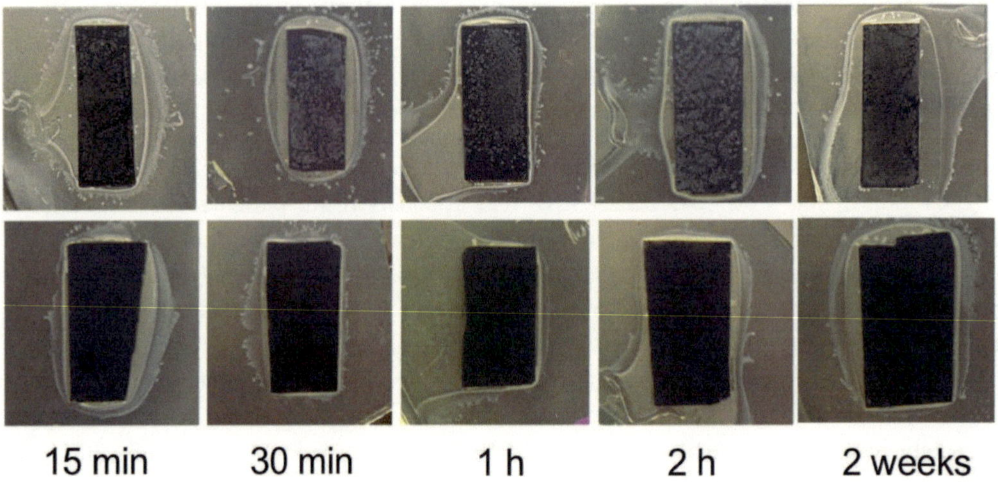

Figure 1. Media-borne assay with *S. aureus* with increasing time of incubation in bacterial solution; top row shows bare substrates completely colonized by bacteria (light beige colored dots); bottom row shows (DMLPEI/PAA)10 films with degradable top films completely eroded with no sign of colonization by bacteria (black colored substrate). From Wong et al., Journal of the American Chemical Society 2010.

3. Conclusion / recommendation

Concerning the severe consequences arising from an infected implanted pacemaker or defibrillator and the data available there should be no discussion on the use of preventive perioperative antibiotics. Randomized data were reported only on the use of a single shot cephfazolin although some other antibiotic agents are supposed to be equally efficient as almost every perioperative device infection is caused by staphylococci or streptococci. In some hospitals with a high rate of methicillin resistant staphylococci vancomycin may be the most proper choice. There is an interesting new approach with coated devices that needs further evaluation.

http://dx.doi.org/10.5772/54203

Author details

Joern Schmitt

University of Giessen and Marburg, Medical Clinic I, Department of Cardiology, Giessen, Germany and Kerckhoff Heart and Thorax Center, Department of Cardiology, Bad Nauheim,, Germany

References

[1] Fuster, V, Ryden, L. E, Cannom, D. S, Crijns, H. J, Curtis, A. B, Ellenbogen, K. A, Halperin, J. L, & Kay, G. N. Le Huezey JY, Lowe JE *et al*: (2011). ACCF/AHA/HRS focused updates incorporated into the ACC/AHA/ESC 2006 guidelines for the management of patients with atrial fibrillation: a report of the American College of Cardiology Foundation/American Heart Association Task Force on practice guidelines. *Circulation* 2011, 123(10):e , 269-367.

[2] Camm AJ, Kirchhof P, Lip GY, Schotten U, Savelieva I, Ernst S, Van Gelder IC, Al-Attar N, Hindricks G, Prendergast B *et al*: Guidelines for the management of atrial fibrillation: the Task Force for the Management of Atrial Fibrillation of the European Society of Cardiology (ESC). *Eur Heart J* 2010, 31(19):2369-2429.

[3] Lip GY, Andreotti F, Fauchier L, Huber K, Hylek E, Knight E, Lane DA, Levi M, Marin F, Palareti G *et al*: Bleeding risk assessment and management in atrial fibrillation patients: a position document from the European Heart Rhythm Association, endorsed by the European Society of Cardiology Working Group on Thrombosis. *Europace* 2011, 13(5):723-746.

[4] Calkins, H, Kuck, K. H, Cappato, R, Brugada, J, Camm, A. J, Chen, S. A, Crijns, H. J, & Damiano, R. J. Jr., Davies DW, DiMarco J *et al*: (2012). HRS/EHRA/ECAS expert consensus statement on catheter and surgical ablation of atrial fibrillation: recommendations for patient selection, procedural techniques, patient management and follow-up, definitions, endpoints, and research trial design: a report of the Heart Rhythm Society (HRS) Task Force on Catheter and Surgical Ablation of Atrial Fibrillation. Developed in partnership with the European Heart Rhythm Association (EHRA), a registered branch of the European Society of Cardiology (ESC) and the European Cardiac Arrhythmia Society (ECAS); and in collaboration with the American College of Cardiology (ACC), American Heart Association (AHA), the Asia Pacific Heart Rhythm Society (APHRS), and the Society of Thoracic Surgeons (STS). Endorsed by the governing bodies of the American College of Cardiology Foundation, the American Heart Association, the European Cardiac Arrhythmia Society, the European Heart Rhythm Association, the Society of Thoracic Surgeons, the Asia Pacific Heart Rhythm Society, and the Heart Rhythm Society. *Heart Rhythm* 2012, 9(4): 632-696 e621.

[5] Tompkins, C. Henrikson CA: Optimal strategies for the management of antiplatelet and anticoagulation medications prior to cardiac device implantation. *Cardiol J* (2011).

[6] Thal, S, Moukabary, T, Boyella, R, Shanmugasundaram, M, Pierce, M. K, & Thai, H. Goldman S: The relationship between warfarin, aspirin, and clopidogrel continuation in the peri-procedural period and the incidence of hematoma formation after device implantation. *Pacing Clin Electrophysiol* (2010).

[7] Tompkins C, Cheng A, Dalal D, Brinker JA, Leng CT, Marine JE, Nazarian S, Spragg DD, Sinha S, Halperin H *et al*: Dual antiplatelet therapy and heparin "bridging" significantly increase the risk of bleeding complications after pacemaker or implantable cardioverter-defibrillator device implantation. *J Am Coll Cardiol* 2010, 55(21): 2376-2382.

[8] Kutinsky, I. B, Jarandilla, R, & Jewett, M. Haines DE: Risk of hematoma complications after device implant in the clopidogrel era. *Circ Arrhythm Electrophysiol* (2010).

[9] Smith, P. K, Goodnough, L. T, Levy, J. H, Poston, R. S, Short, M. A, & Weerakkody, G. J. Lenarz LA: Mortality Benefit With Prasugrel in the TRITON-TIMI 38 Coronary Artery Bypass Grafting Cohort: Risk-Adjusted Retrospective Data Analysis. *J Am Coll Cardiol* (2012).

[10] Wiviott SD, Braunwald E, McCabe CH, Montalescot G, Ruzyllo W, Gottlieb S, Neumann FJ, Ardissino D, De Servi S, Murphy SA *et al*: Prasugrel versus clopidogrel in patients with acute coronary syndromes. *N Engl J Med* 2007, 357(20):2001-2015.

[11] Montalescot, G, Wiviott, S. D, Braunwald, E, Murphy, S. A, Gibson, C. M, & Mccabe, C. H. Antman EM: Prasugrel compared with clopidogrel in patients undergoing percutaneous coronary intervention for ST-elevation myocardial infarction (TRITON-TIMI 38): double-blind, randomised controlled trial. *Lancet* (2009).

[12] Becker RC, Bassand JP, Budaj A, Wojdyla DM, James SK, Cornel JH, French J, Held C, Horrow J, Husted S *et al*: Bleeding complications with the P2Y12 receptor antagonists clopidogrel and ticagrelor in the PLATelet inhibition and patient Outcomes (PLATO) trial. *Eur Heart J* 2011, 32(23):2933-2944.

[13] Cannon CP, Harrington RA, James S, Ardissino D, Becker RC, Emanuelsson H, Husted S, Katus H, Keltai M, Khurmi NS *et al*: Comparison of ticagrelor with clopidogrel in patients with a planned invasive strategy for acute coronary syndromes (PLATO): a randomised double-blind study. *Lancet* 2010, 375(9711):283-293.

[14] Hoffmeister, H. M, Bode, C, Darius, H, Huber, K, Rybak, K, & Silber, S. Unterbrechung antithrombotischer Behandlung (Bridging) bei kardialen Erkrankunen. Positionspapier. *Kardiologe* (2010).

[15] Giudici, M. C. Barold SS: Device implantation and anticoagulation. *J Interv Cardiol* (2002).

[16] Wiegand, U. K. LeJeune D, Boguschewski F, Bonnemeier H, Eberhardt F, Schunkert H, Bode F: Pocket hematoma after pacemaker or implantable cardioverter defibrillator surgery: influence of patient morbidity, operation strategy, and perioperative antiplatelet/anticoagulation therapy. *Chest* (2004).

[17] Ghanbari, H, Feldman, D, Schmidt, M, Ottino, J, Machado, C, Akoum, N, & Wall, T. S. Daccarett M: Cardiac resynchronization therapy device implantation in patients with therapeutic international normalized ratios. *Pacing Clin Electrophysiol* (2010).

[18] Healey JS, Eikelboom J, Douketis J, Wallentin L, Oldgren J, Yang S, Themeles E, Heidbuchle H, Avezum A, Reilly P *et al*: Periprocedural Bleeding and Thromboembolic Events With Dabigatran Compared With Warfarin: Results From the Randomized Evaluation of Long-Term Anticoagulation Therapy (RE-LY) Randomized Trial. *Circulation* 2012, 126(3):343-348.

[19] Friedman, R. J, Kurth, A, Clemens, A, Noack, H, & Eriksson, B. I. Caprini JA: Dabigatran etexilate and concomitant use of non-steroidal anti-inflammatory drugs or acetylsalicylic acid in patients undergoing total hip and total knee arthroplasty: No increased risk of bleeding. *Thromb Haemost* (2012).

[20] Bernard, M. L, Shotwell, M, & Nietert, P. J. Gold MR: Meta-analysis of bleeding complications associated with cardiac rhythm device implantation. *Circ Arrhythm Electrophysiol* (2012).

[21] Korantzopoulos, P, Letsas, K. P, Liu, T, Fragakis, N, & Efremidis, M. Goudevenos JA: Anticoagulation and antiplatelet therapy in implantation of electrophysiological devices. *Europace* (2011).

[22] Hill PE: Complications of permanent transvenous cardiac pacing: a year review of all transvenous pacemakers inserted at one community hospital *Pacing Clin Electrophysiol* (1987). Pt 1):564-570.

[23] Frame, R, Brodman, R. F, Furman, S, & Andrews, C. A. Gross JN: Surgical removal of infected transvenous pacemaker leads. *Pacing Clin Electrophysiol* (1993).

[24] Voigt, A, & Shalaby, A. Saba S: Continued rise in rates of cardiovascular implantable electronic device infections in the United States: temporal trends and causative insights. *Pacing Clin Electrophysiol* (2010).

[25] Sohail, M. R, Uslan, D. Z, Khan, A. H, Friedman, P. A, Hayes, D. L, Wilson, W. R, Steckelberg, J. M, & Stoner, S. M. Baddour LM: Risk factor analysis of permanent pacemaker infection. *Clin Infect Dis* (2007).

[26] Darouiche, R. O, & Wall, M. J. Jr., Itani KM, Otterson MF, Webb AL, Carrick MM, Miller HJ, Awad SS, Crosby CT, Mosier MC *et al*: Chlorhexidine-Alcohol versus Povidone-Iodine for Surgical-Site Antisepsis. *N Engl J Med* (2010).

[27] Da Costa AKirkorian G, Cucherat M, Delahaye F, Chevalier P, Cerisier A, Isaaz K, Touboul P: Antibiotic prophylaxis for permanent pacemaker implantation: a meta-analysis. *Circulation* (1998).

[28] Matl, F. D, Zlotnyk, J, Obermeier, A, Friess, W, Vogt, S, Buchner, H, Schnabelrauch, H, & Stemberger, A. Kuhn KD: New anti-infective coatings of surgical sutures based on a combination of antiseptics and fatty acids. *J Biomater Sci Polym Ed* (2009).

[29] Wong, S. Y, Moskowitz, J. S, Veselinovic, J, Rosario, R. A, Timachova, K, Blaisse, M. R, Fuller, R. C, & Klibanov, A. M. Hammond PT: Dual functional polyelectrolyte multilayer coatings for implants: permanent microbicidal base with controlled release of therapeutic agents. *J Am Chem Soc* (2010).

[30] Bertaglia, E, Zerbo, F, Zardo, S, Barzan, D, & Zoppo, F. Pascotto P: Antibiotic prophylaxis with a single dose of cephazolin during pacemaker implantation: incidence of long-term infective complications. *Pacing Clin Electrophysiol* (2006).

[31] Ferguson, T. B. Jr., Ferguson CL, Crites K, Crimmins-Reda P: The additional hospital costs generated in the management of complications of pacemaker and defibrillator implantations. *J Thorac Cardiovasc Surg* (1996). discussion , 751-742.

[32] Darouiche RO: Treatment of infections associated with surgical implants. (2004). *N Engl J Med*, .

[33] Dababneh, A. S. Sohail MR: Cardiovascular implantable electronic device infection: a stepwise approach to diagnosis and management. *Cleve Clin J Med* (2011).

[34] Maytin, M. Epstein LM: Proof positive: efficacy of antibiotic prophylaxis in device implantation. *Circ Arrhythm Electrophysiol* (2009).

[35] Bluhm, G, & Jacobson, B. Ransjo U: Antibiotic prophylaxis in pacemaker surgery: a prospective trial with local or systemic administration of antibiotics at generator replacements. *Pacing Clin Electrophysiol* (1985).

[36] De Oliveira, J. C, Martinelli, M, Nishioka, S. A, Varejao, T, Uipe, D, Pedrosa, A. A, Costa, R, Avila, D, & Danik, A. SB: Efficacy of antibiotic prophylaxis before the implantation of pacemakers and cardioverter-defibrillators: results of a large, prospective, randomized, double-blinded, placebo-controlled trial. *Circ Arrhythm Electrophysiol* (2009).

[37] Tarakji, K. G, Chan, E. J, Cantillon, D. J, Doonan, A. L, Hu, T, Schmitt, S, Fraser, T. G, Kim, A, & Gordon, S. M. Wilkoff BL: Cardiac implantable electronic device infections: presentation, management, and patient outcomes. *Heart Rhythm* (2010).

[38] Sohail, M. R, Uslan, D. Z, Khan, A. H, Friedman, P. A, Hayes, D. L, Wilson, W. R, Steckelberg, J. M, & Stoner, S. Baddour LM: Management and outcome of permanent pacemaker and implantable cardioverter-defibrillator infections. *J Am Coll Cardiol* (2007).

Chapter 8

Defibrillator Threshold Testing

Munir Zaqqa

Additional information is available at the end of the chapter

http://dx.doi.org/10.5772/52594

1. Introduction

Since implantable cardioverter-defibrillators (ICDs) were first introduced, defibrillator threshold (DFT) testing was considered an integral part of the implant procedure. Performing DFT testing verifies the ability of the ICD in detecting and aborting the lethal arrhythmia it was designed to treat. The process has evolved with the development of the ICD's and the expanding indications for their usage. Recent studies even questioned the need for DFT assessment. Currently this matter is controversial with no firm guidelines. In this chapter we present the basic information on DFT testing, how to manage high DFT, and then discuss the evidence for and against performing the test.

2. DFT concept

DFT testing is performed by inducing ventricular arrhythmia and then finding the minimal amount of energy delivered by the ICD to defibrillate the myocardium back to sinus rhythm. Central to the concept of determining the DFT, was the discovery since 1930, that electrical shocks themselves can induce ventricular fibrillation (VF) [1]. By giving a shock during the vulnerable period of repolarization, VF could be reproducibly induced. Ventricular tachycardia (VT) may also be induced, but in a relatively small percentage of patients [2]. As the amount of energy delivered during the vulnerable period is increased, a threshold is reached that does not induce VF [3]. This is called the upper limit of vulnerability (ULV) and is proportional to DFT value [4-5]. This concept can be used as a surrogate for DFT [6-7]. Instead of inducing VF and checking the threshold at which it terminates, a different protocol is used that delivers variable strengths of shocks during the vulnerable T-wave phase and then establishes ULV. As compared to regular DFT test, ULV test is done during sinus rhythm and not during VF. Using this approach there is a need for more number of shocks, but less number of times that VF are induced.

The threshold to terminate ventricular fibrillation with ICD's is usually in the 5 to 30 J range. It was the ability to reduce the energy requirements by 10 folds as compared to external defibrillator that made the ICD a reality [8]. Otherwise the size of the ICD would have to be much bigger to store the needed energy for defibrillation. Although the threshold is expressed in relation to the energy discharged by the ICD, in reality it is the voltage and its duration that is the critical factor in defibrillation [9-10]. Duration has a relatively narrow range to be effective (in the range of few milliseconds). To achieve this precise phase duration of defibrillation, the capacitor discharge is truncated in either a tilt based formula which truncates the discharge after a certain percentage of decay in the voltage has been reached, or more simply in a time based manner after a certain time has elapsed. Voltage is usually in the hundreds of volts range. If voltage is too low it may induce rather than terminate fibrillation as explained earlier. High voltage (above 1000 Volts) is also not without its risks, as it may result in stunning of the myocardium and subsequent electromechanical dissociation [11-12]. The voltage wave form can be manipulated to make defibrillation more effective and therefore require less energy. Biphasic wave, which is the standard now in ICD's, has reversal of the initial polarity. The initial wave results in charging of the cell membrane as a result of the voltage gradient. The reversal which is termed "burping" is theorized to absorb the initial energy and therefore avoid proarrhythmia [11-12]. The biphasic wave form can be manipulated by changing the initial voltage, and by changing the duration and the ratio of its waves. Different manufactures use different formulas in their devices, and some allow changing of the parameters by the electrophysiologists in case of high DFT.

3. Performing DFT testing

Before doing DFT testing, consent should be taken from the patient explaining the risk and benefit of the procedure. Vital signs should be stable and basic lab results such as electrolytes should be within normal range. There should be no contraindication to performing the test such as severe aortic stenosis or intracavitary thrombus. An external defibrillator should be placed ready next to the patient, preferably with defibrillator patches attached to the patient. As the shock is painful, adequate sedation or short anesthesia should be given with careful monitoring of vital signs and saturation level [14].

After the device is implanted good lead position should be verified by X-ray. The lead is tested to ensure adequate sensing and pacing thresholds and normal impedance values.

Prior to VF induction, the device is activated and programmed with the amount of energy to be delivered. Ventricular fibrillation is usually induced via the device. There are several methods of VF induction such as programmed ventricular stimulation, T wave shock, fast burst pacing, or by applying low voltage direct current [15]. Following VF induction the patient is monitored carefully until the device detects the arrhythmia and restores it back to sinus rhythm. If the device fails, external defibrillation should be immediately performed.

To find the exact DFT value, this process has to be repeated several times with either a step up, step down, or a binary fashion until DFT or ULV are found [16-17]. Although the term threshold should indicate a value above which defibrillation is successful and below which shocks fail, in reality DFT is a probabilistic phenomenon with a certain percentage of success rate [17-18]. One shock may be successful while a successive one with the same conditions may fail [5]. Despite the poor reproducibility of DFT, it is still a useful parameter, as this value taken with a safety margin above it, gives a high clinical success of VF termination. The standard safety margin is 10 J, although 5 J may be enough [19-20].

DFT testing with several shocks and titrations may be useful in a research protocol, where the exact value has important clinical significance. A simpler, yet safe approach is the defibrillator safety margin (DSM) test [21]. In this method, a single or two VF inductions may be enough. The device is usually programmed to a value that is expected to restore sinus rhythm following induction. This value depends on the operator preference. It is usually an average value that is at least 10 J below the maximum output of the device [22]. If it is successful, then this value should at least be equal to the DFT value. If the shock fails, then step up approach has to be used to find the threshold.

Study	Year	N	Percent
Kelly et al [23]	1988	94	5.3%
Winkle et al [24]	1989	270	2.6%
Pinski et al [25]	1991	125	18%
Epstein et al [26]	1992	1946	4.6%
Gold et al [27]	1997	114	8%
Brodsky et al [28]	1999	764	3.1%
Shukla et al [29]	2003	968	11%
Russo et al [30]	2005	1139	6.2%
Theuns et al [31]	2005	127	14%
Mainigi et al [32]	2006	121	12%
Guenther et al [33]	2012	975	1.4%
Cheng et al [34]	2012	243	5.3%

Table 1. Incidence of high DFT

High DFT, defined in most studies as a threshold of < 10 J below the maximum output of the device, is estimated to occur in about 5% of ICD implants (range 1.4 to 18%) (Tables 1) [23-33]. Although the exact value of DFT cannot be predicted in an individual patient prior to testing, there are some clinical parameters associated with increased thresholds (Table 2) [27-29,32-35].

Young age
Low ejection fraction
Hypertrophic cardiomyopathy
Non coronary artery disease
Medications (specially amiodarone)
Larger and small left ventricular sizes
Large body size
Prolonged QRS duration

Table 2. Clinical factors associated with high DFT 's

DFT testing is usually performed introperatively at the time of implant before the pocket is closed to allow intervention in case of high thresholds. Sometimes it is done at the time of discharge or at a later time when the lead has assumed a stable position [28,36].

4. Management of high DFT

If a patient is found to have elevated thresholds, the initial step is to verify that this is not caused by a reversible problem related to the implant procedure itself (table 3). If no reversible cause is found, then there are several options available. These are classified into non-invasive and invasive methods (table 4).

Hypotension
Pneumothorax
Pericardial effusion
Large pleural effusion
Pulmonary edema
Sedation related such as aspiration and hypoxia
Acidosis
Electrolyte imbalance
Medications
Ischemia
Prolonged procedure
Lead dislodgment

Table 3. Reversible causes of high DFT

Adjustment to improve DFT	Comment
Non Invasive	
Medications [37-41]	Particularly amiodarone has been shown to increase thresholds. Medications that potentially decrease thresholds include sotalol and dofetilide.
Lead Polarity [43-44]	The RV lead is the anode (positive) vector. It may be changed to cathode (negative).
Vector of defibrillation [41,45]	Adding an SVC coil is most effective when a single coil has high resistance of > 58 ohm. If dual coil system is implanted, the vector can be changed electronically.
Wave form [41,46]	Change of Tilt and phase duration of shocks is available in some devices and may be optimized individually.
Invasive	
Lead repositioning [47-48]	Apical position has lower DFT when compared to a proximal position. Septal and RVOT positions may have lower thresholds
Addition of extra leads to change the vector of the shock [49-51].	Subcutaneous array, coronary sinus and azygous vein leads could be introduced to lower thresholds
Upgrading to higher output device	

Table 4. Approaches to improve DFT

Changing or stopping a medication associated with high threshold may help the problem [37]. Amiodarone has been particularly quoted in the literature as causing high thresholds [38]. Other possible medications include lidocaine and verapamil. On the other hand, medications that do not affect or potentially reduce DFT include sotalol, dofetilide, beta-blocker and dronedarone [37-40].

There are some programmable parameters in the ICD that can affect DFT. These include polarity of the lead, the vector of defibrillation, and the tilt and duration of the shock wave [41-42]. The lead is configured with an anodal (positive) distal coil. This configuration results in an average reduction of 15% in DFT as compared to a cathodal right ventricular (RV) coil [43]. Reversing it to cathode results in the energy propagating away from the lead instead of "collapsing" towards it. This is theorized to increase the arrhythmia potential. However, changing polarity has been shown to decrease DFT in some of the patients and this configuration can therefore be attempted [44].

A dual-coil, active pectoral lead system is the most commonly used configuration. A proximal coil placed in the superior vena cava (SVC) area has been found to decrease DFT as compared to a single coil system [41,45]. This effect is particularly effective when the single coil resistance is high (above 58 ohm), while the effect on the threshold is mixed with low single coil resistance. Control of proximal coil can be done electronically in a dual coil lead. Addition of an SVC coil might be considered in patients with single coil and high resistance.

The proximal coil location should be in the high SVC and brachiocephalic area rather than the low SVC and atrial area as the later is associated with higher DFT value [45].

The phase duration of defibrillation is critical in achieving sinus rhythm [9-10]. The optimal phase duration is not exactly known and it can be optimized in some devices for individual patients with high DFT's [46].

Changing a nominal parameter should not be taken lightly, as these are the ones tested and proven with clinical research. Any adjustment made to the settings should be verified by repeated induction and the reassurance of a successful defibrillation.

Several invasive choices that reduce DFT are available. Changing the RV lead location may reduce DFT. The standard RV position is the RV apex. This has the advantage of a stable position and good threshold. Alternative lead positions that have good thresholds are the right ventricular outflow tract (RVOT) and the septum. An active fixation system should be used in these areas. A right free wall position has the highest DFT [47-48]. Changing the shock vector may lower DFT. This can be achieved by incorporating subcutaneous array or an additional lead in the azygous vein or the coronary sinus [49-51]. Upgrading to higher output devices may be useful in patients with borderline elevated thresholds.

5. The arguments for and against performing DFT testing

Since implanting ICD's in the early 1980's, VF induction and testing the device ability to restore sinus rhythm not only helped in determining DFT's, but also allowed testing of the sensing capability of the device, the ability of the programmed algorithm to recognize the arrhythmia, and the ability of the capacitors to deliver the stored energy. This was an important step in testing a new device that is designed to treat a lethal arrhythmia. Patients who were found to have high threshold had intervention performed to attempt to lower the DFT's. If the thresholds could not be lowered then many physicians did not implant the device. This was because of the concern that a shock might change a stable VT into VF and then not be able to terminate it. There were several reports of increased mortality in patients with high DFT and case reports of deaths due to failed defibrillation. [23,28,52-54] (table 5). Intuitively, finding DFT will result in reduced mortality as it allows the recognition of patients who will not respond to the shock and therefore find a subgroup of patients who need further intervention. However, this matter is not so simple.

Testing involves induction of ventricular fibrillation in patients with significant heart disease with a potential for morbidity and mortality. Complications associates with DFT testing include worsening heart failure, hemodynamic compromise, cerebrovascular accidents and even deaths. In the Canadian Experience study by Bernie et al which looked at 19,067 patients, thirty five patients (0.18%) had serious complications [61]. The recognition of the complications was coupled with improvements in the lead and defibrillator technology. In addition, ICD use expanded considerably after studies showed its benefit not only in secondary but also in primary prevention of sudden death. This changed the risk benefit ratio of

DFT testing. Several studies gradually emerged that questioned the need to find DFT (table 5). This lack of benefit of DFT testing shown in several studies may be explained by several factors:

- The comparison of the mortality in patients who had DFT testing versus those who did not have a test may be a biased by excluding unstable patients from DFT testing and including them in the non tested group.
- The comparison should include the morbidity and mortality associated with the test itself and also the problems related to the intervention to reduce DFT. Even simple measures such as changing a medication and reprogramming the ICD could have an impact on mortality, not to mention possible complications associated with invasive interventions. The shock itself done during the test may have an impact on patients with established cardiac disease. Defibrillation has been shown to increase troponin level [62]. Any shock, even when inappropriate, has been associated with increased mortality [63].
- DFT does not predict future successful defibrillation in a reliable manner [18]. This may be related to the probabilistic nature of the test. It has also been shown that DFT change acutely and chronically [64-65]. This could result in the improvement of high DFT, but may also result in a patient with normal DFT developing high thresholds with time. It is estimated that about 29% of deaths in ICD recipients are still due to arrhythmias that could not be terminated by the ICD [66].
- Ventricular fibrillation induced in the hospital is not the same as the real world arrhythmia. Induced VF tends to be more organized than spontaneous VF [67]. In the clinical setting, many patients have ventricular tachycardia rather than VF or even do not have any arrhythmia at all during the lifetime of the implant [2,68-69]. For these patients DFT test may be misleading or may not have any relevance at all.

It is therefore important to have to prospective randomized study to give us a clear answer. One prospective, but not randomized study (SAFE-ICD) showed no benefit of DFT testing [60]. The result of an ongoing study (SIMPLE trial) may give a more clear direction once finished [70].

The approach to DFT testing has changed over time. A recent study in 111 Italian centers over the period 2007 to 2010 involving 2,082 patients documented the trend change [71]. It reported DFT testing to be performed in 38% of patients with the incidence declining annually from 36% in 2007 to 28% in 2010. In 13% of centers, the test was performed routinely, and in 38% it was not performed at all. The reasons for not performing DFT testing in this survey were the policy of the center in 44%, a primary indication for the implant in 31% and doing a device replacement in 15%. Not doing DFT testing can certainly make the ICD implant simpler. The simplification is not just related to the procedure itself, but starts with the initial step of taking the consent from the patient. It is not a simple task to explain the risk to the patient in a lay term without confusing him. A physician has to explain that after the surgery has finished successfully, there will be a need to stop the heart; and that there is a chance, even though very small, that he may have a problem like stroke or that we may not be able to restore his heart to beat back again.

Author	Year	N	Comment
Favor DFT testing			
Marchlinski et al [54]	1988	33	Patients with low DFT (n=19) had 100% success rate of clinical arrhythmia termination as compared to 73% (n=14) in the high threshold group
Pires et al [22]	2006	835	Long term survival was lower in the no DFT testing group (n=203) in comparison to DFT and safety margin testing (n=632)
Hall et al [55]	2007	112	Higher mortality seen in patients who did not have DFT testing because of contraindication (n=55) as compared to a random sample who had DFT testing performed (n=57)
Against DFT testing			
Epstein et al [26]	1992	1946	There was improved mortality among patients with high DFT who received ICD (n=71) versus those who did not receive ICD (n=16)
Russo et al [30]	2005	1139	No difference in mortality among patients with high DFT who had intervention (n=34) versus who did not have intervention (n=37)
Blatt et al [56]	2008	717	No difference in mortality between lower (< or =10 J) (n=547) versus higher (n=170) DFT groups
Bianchi et al [57]	2009	291	No difference in mortality between Italian centers that perform DFT testing routinely (n=137) versus centers that do not perform DFT testing (n=154)
Michowitz et al [58]	2011	256	No difference in mortality between CRT-D patient who had DFT testing (n=204) versus who did not have DFT testing (n=52)
Codner et al [59]	2012	213	No difference in mortality between DFT testing (n=80) and no DFT testing (n=133) groups
Brignole et al [60]	2012	2120	Prospective but non randomized evaluation of DFT testing (n=836) versus no DFT testing (n=1284) showed no difference in mortality

Table 5. Studies favoring and against DFT testing.

6. Conclusion

The approach to DFT testing has changed since ICD's were first introduced. It has changed from being an essential part performed in all the patients to being done in less than one third of the patients at current time. The need for DFT testing is a balance between benefit and risk with studies showing conflicting results. Most recent studies show equal benefit risk ratio for DFT testing. A prospective randomized study is needed to resolve the issue and there is currently one being performed. When this study is finished it should give a more clear answer regarding this issue.

Author details

Munir Zaqqa*

Address all correspondence to: munirzaqqa@yahoo.com

Jordan University Hospital, Jordan

References

[1] Wiggers, C. J., & Wegria, R. (1940). Ventricular fibrillation due to single, localized induction and condenser shocks applied during the vulnerable phase of ventricular systole. *Am J Physiol*, 128, 500-505.

[2] Zima, E., Gergely, M., Soós, P., et al. (2006). The effect of induction method on defibrillation threshold and ventricular fibrillation cycle length. *J Cardiovasc Electrophysiol.*, Apr, 17(4), 377-81.

[3] Yashima, M., Kim, Y. H., Armin, S., et al. (2003). On the mechanism of the probabilistic nature of ventricular defibrillation threshold. *Am J Physiol Heart Circ Physiol.*, Jan, 284(1), H249-55.

[4] Day, J. D., Doshi, R. N., Belott, P., Birgersdotter, , et al. (2007). Inductionless or limited shock testing is possible in most patients with implantable cardioverter- defibrillators/cardiac resynchronization therapy defibrillators: results of the multicenter ASSURE Study (Arrhythmia Single Shock Defibrillation Threshold Testing Versus Upper Limit of Vulnerability: Risk Reduction Evaluation With Implantable Cardioverter-Defibrillator Implantations). *Circulation.*, May 8;, 115(18), 2382-9.

[5] Swerdlow, C. D., Davie, S., Ahern, T., et al. (1996). Comparative reproducibility of defibrillation threshold and upper limit of vulnerability. *Pacing Clin Electrophysiol.*, Dec, 19(12 Pt 1), 2103-11.

[6] Hwang, C., Swerdlow, C. D., Kass, R. M., et al. (1994). Upper limit of vulnerability reliably predicts the defibrillation threshold in humans. *Circulation.*, Nov, 90(5), 2308-14.

[7] Swerdlow, C. D., Ahern, T., Kass, R. M., et al. (1996). Upper limit of vulnerability is a good estimator of shock strength associated with 90% probability of successful defibrillation in humans with transvenous implantable cardioverter-defibrillators. *J Am Coll Cardiol.*, Apr, 27(5), 1112-8.

[8] Mirowski, M., Mower, M. M., Reid, P. R., et al. (1982). The automatic implantable defibrillator. New Modality for treatment of life-threatening ventricular arrhythmias. *Pacing Clin Electrophysiol.*, May, 5(3), 384-401.

[9] Kroll, M. W., & Swerdlow, C. D. (2007). Optimizing defibrillation waveforms for ICDs. J Interv Card Electrophysiol.Apr Epub 2007 Jun 1. Review. , 18(3), 247-63.

[10] Jacob, S., Pidlaoan, V., Singh, J., et al. (2010). High defibrillation threshold: the science, signs and solutions. *Indian Pacing Electrophysiol J.*, Jan 7, 10(1), 21-39.

[11] Mitchell, L. B., Pineda, E. A., et al. (2002). Sudden death in patients with implantable cardioverter defibrillators: The importance of post-shock electromechanical dissociation. *Journal of the American College of Cardiology*, 39, 1323-1328.

[12] Xie, J., Weil, M. H., Sun, S., et al. (1997). High-energy defibrillation increases the severity of postresuscitation myocardial dysfunction. CirculationJul 15; , 96(2), 683-8.

[13] Swerdlow, C. D., Fan, W., & Brewer, J. E. (1996). Charge-burping theory correctly predicts optimal ratios of phase duration for biphasic defibrillation waveforms. *Circulation.*, Nov 1, 94(9), 2278-84.

[14] Marquié, C., Duchemin, A., Klug, D., et al. (2007). Can we implant cardioverter defibrillator under minimal sedation? *Europace.*, Jul, 9(7), 545-50.

[15] Euler, D. E., Whitman, T. A., Roberts, P. R., et al. (1999). Low voltage direct current delivered through unipolar transvenous leads: an alternate method for the induction of ventricular fibrillation. *Pacing Clin Electrophysiol.*, Jun, 22(6 Pt 1), 908-14.

[16] Shorofsky, S. R., Peters, R. W., Rashba, E. J., et al. (2004). Comparison of step-down and binary search algorithms for determination of defibrillation threshold in humans. *Pacing Clin Electrophysiol.*, Feb, 27(2), 218-20.

[17] Swerdlow, C. D., Russo, A. M., & Degroot, P. J. (2007). The dilemma of ICD implant testing. Pacing Clin Electrophysiol.May Review., 30(5), 675-700.

[18] Degroot, P. J., Church, T. R., Mehra, R., et al. (1997). Derivation of a defibrillator implant criterion based on probability of successful defibrillation. *Pacing Clin Electrophysiol.*, Aug, 20(8 Pt 1), 924-35.

[19] Marchlinski, F. E., Flores, B., Miller, J. M., et al. (1988). Relation of the intraoperative defibrillation threshold to successful postoperative defibrillation with an automatic implantable cardioverter defibrillator. *Am J Cardiol.*, Sep 1, 62(7), 393-8.

[20] Gold, M. R., Higgins, S., Klein, R., et al. (2002). Efficacy and temporal stability of reduced safety margins for ventricular defibrillation: primary results from the Low Energy Safety Study (LESS). *Circulation.*, Apr 30, 105(17), 2043-8.

[21] Higgins, S., Mann, D., Calkins, H., et al. (2005). One conversion of ventricular fibrillation is adequate for implantable cardioverter-debibrillator implant: An analysis from the low energy safety study (LESS). *Heart Rhythm*, 2, 117-22.

[22] Pires, L. A. (2007). Defibrillation testing of the implantable cardioverter defibrillator: when, how, and by whom? *Indian Pacing Electrophysiol J.*, Aug 1, 7(3), 166-75.

[23] Kelly, P. A., Cannom, D. S., Garan, H., et al. (1988). The automatic implantable cardioverter-defibrillator: efficacy, complications and survival in patients with malignant ventricular arrhythmias. *J Am Coll Cardiol.*, Jun, 11(6), 1278-86.

[24] Winkle, R. A., Mead, R. H., Ruder, M. A., et al. (1989). Long-term outcome with the automatic implantable cardioverter-defibrillator. *J Am Coll Cardiol.*, May, 13(6), 1353-61.

[25] Pinski, S. L., Vanerio, G., Castle, L. W., et al. (1991). Patients with a high defibrillation threshold: Clinical characteristics, management, and outcome. *Am Heart J*, 122(1 Pt 1), 89-95.

[26] Epstein, A. E., Ellenbogen, K. A., Kirk, K. A., et al. (1992). Clinical characteristics and outcome of patients with high defibrillation thresholds. *A multicenter study. Circulation.*, Oct, 86(4), 1206-16.

[27] Gold, M. R., Khalighi, K., Kavesh, N. G., et al. (1997). Clinical predictors of transvenous biphasic defibrillation thresholds. *Am J Cardiol.*, Jun 15, 79(12), 1623-7.

[28] Brodsky, C. M., Chang, F., & Vlay, S. C. (1999). Multicenter evaluation of implantable cardioverter defibrillator testing after implant: the Post Implant Testing Study (PITS). *Pacing Clin Electrophysiol.*, Dec, 22(12), 1769-76.

[29] Shukla, H. H., Flaker, G. C., Jayam, V., et al. (2003). High defibrillation thresholds in transvenous biphasic implantable defibrillators: clinical predictors and prognostic implications. *Pacing Clin Electrophysiol.*, Jan, 26(1 Pt 1), 44-8.

[30] Russo, A. M., Sauer, W., Gerstenfeld, E. P., et al. (2005). Defibrillation threshold testing: is it really necessary at the time of implantable cardioverter-defibrillator insertion? *Heart Rhythm.*, May, 2(5), 456-61.

[31] Theuns, D. A., Szili-Torok, T., & Jordaens, L. J. (2005). Defibrillation efficacy testing: long-term follow-up and mortality. *Europace.*, Nov, 7(6), 509-15.

[32] Mainigi, S. K., Cooper, J. M., Russo, A. M., et al. (2006). Elevated defibrillation thresholds in patients undergoing biventricular defibrillator implantation: incidence and predictors. Heart Rhythm.Sep , 3(9), 1010-6.

[33] Guenther, M., Rauwolf, T., Brüggemann, B., & Gerlach, . (2012). Pre-hospital discharge testing after implantable cardioverter defibrillator implantation: a measure of safety or out of date? A retrospective analysis of 975 patients. *Europace*, Feb, 14(2), 217-23.

[34] Cheng, Z., Turakhia, M., Lo, R., et al. (2012). Incidence and clinical predictors of low defibrillation safety margin at time of implantable defibrillator implantation. *J Interv Card Electrophysiol.*, Jun, 34(1), 93-100.

[35] Quin, E. M., Cuoco, F. A., Forcina, M. S., et al. (2011). Defibrillation thresholds in hypertrophic cardiomyopathy. *J Cardiovasc Electrophysiol.*, May, 22(5), 569-72.

[36] Goldberger, J. J., Horvath, G., Inbar, S., et al. (1997). Utility of predischarge and one-month transvenous implantable defibrillator tests. *Am J Cardiol*, 79, 822e6.

[37] Dopp, A. L., Miller, J. M., & Tisdale, J. E. (2008). Effect of drugs on defibrillation capacity. *Drugs*, 68(5), 607-30, Review.

[38] Hohnloser, S. H., Dorian, P., Roberts, R., et al. (2006). Effect of amiodarone and sotalol on ventricular defibrillation threshold: the optimal pharmacological therapy in cardioverter defibrillator patients (OPTIC) trial. *Circulation*, Jul 11, 114(2), 104-9.

[39] Simon, R. D., Sturdivant, J. L., Leman, R. B., et al. (2009). The effect of dofetilide on ventricular defibrillation thresholds. *Pacing Clin Electrophysiol.*, Jan, 32(1), 24-8.

[40] Chevalier, P., Timour, Q., Morel, E., et al. (2012). Chronic oral amiodarone but not dronedarone therapy increases ventricular defibrillation threshold during acute myocardial ischemia in a closed-chest animal model. *J Cardiovasc Pharmacol.*, Jun, 59(6), 523-8.

[41] Kroll, M. W., & Schwab, J. O. (2010). Achieving low defibrillation thresholds at implant: pharmacological influences, RV coil polarity and position, SVC coil usage and positioning, pulse width settings, and the azygous vein. Fundam Clin Pharmacol. Oct; 10.1111/j.1472-8206.2010.00848.x.Review, 24(5), 561-73.

[42] Jacob, S., Pidlaoan, V., Singh, J., et al. (2010). High defibrillation threshold: the science, signs and solutions. *Indian Pacing Electrophysiol J.*, Jan 7, 10(1), 21-39.

[43] Olsovsky, M. R., Shorofsky, S. R., & Gold, M. R. (1998). Effect of shock polarity on biphasic defibrillation thresholds using an active pectoral lead system. *J Cardiovasc Electrophysiol.*, Apr, 9(4), 350-4.

[44] Zienciuk, A., Lubiński, A., Królak, T., et al. (2007). Effects of shock polarity reversal on defibrillation threshold in an implantable cardioverter-defibrillator. *Kardiol Pol.*, May, 65(5), 495-500.

[45] Gold, M., Val-Mejias, J., Leman, R. B., et al. (2008). Optimization of superior vena cava coil position and usage for transvenous defibrillation. *Heart Rhythm*, 5-394.

[46] Denman, R. A., Umesan, C., Martin, P. T., et al. (2006). Benefit of millisecond waveform durations for patients with high defibrillation thresholds. *Heart Rhythm*, May, 3(5), 536-41.

[47] Crossley, G. H., Boyce, K., Roelke, M., et al. (2009). A prospective randomized trial of defibrillation thresholds from the right ventricular outflow tract and the right ventricular apex. *Pacing Clin Electrophysiol.*, Feb, 32(2), 166-71.

[48] Yang, F., & Patterson, R. (2008). Optimal transvenous coil position on active-can single-coil ICD defibrillation efficacy: a simulation study. *Ann Biomed Eng*, 36, 1659-67.

[49] Kuhlkamp, V., Dornberger, V., Mewis, C., et al. (2001). Comparison of the efficacy of a subcutaneous array electrode with a subcutaneous patch electrode, a prospective randomized study. *Int. J. Cardiol.*, 78-247.

[50] Seow, S. C., Tolentino, C. S., Zhao, J., et al. (2011). Azygous vein coil lowers defibrillation threshold in patients with high defibrillation threshold. *Europace*, Jun, 13(6), 825-8.

[51] Faheem, O., Padala, A., Kluger, J., et al. (2010). Coronary sinus shocking lead as salvage in patients with advanced CHF and high defibrillation thresholds. *Pacing Clin Electrophysiol.*, Aug, 33(8), 967-72.

[52] Lehmann, M. H., Thomas, A., Nabih, M., et al. (1994). Sudden death in recipients of first generation implantable cardioverter defibrillators: Analysis of terminal events. *Participating investigators. J Interv Cardiol*, 7(5), 487-503.

[53] Winkle, R. A., Mead, R. H., & Ruder, M. A. Gaudiani. (1989). Long-term outcome with the automatic implantable cardioverter-defibrillator. *J Am Coll Cardiol.*, May, 13(6), 1353-61.

[54] Marchlinski, F. E., Flores, B., Miller, J. M., et al. (1988). Relation of the intraoperative defibrillation threshold to successful postoperative defibrillation with an automatic implantable cardioverter defibrillator. *Am J Cardiol.*, Sep 1, 62(7), 393-8.

[55] Hall, B., Jeevanantham, V., Levine, E., et al. (2007). Comparison of outcomes in patients undergoing defibrillation threshold testing at the time of implantable cardioverter-defibrillator implantation versus no defibrillation threshold testing. *Cardiol J*, 14(5), 463-9.

[56] Blatt, J. A., Poole, J. E., Johnson, G. W., et al. (2008). SCD-HeFT Investigators. No benefit from defibrillation threshold testing in the SCD-HeFT (Sudden Cardiac Death in Heart Failure Trial). *J Am Coll Cardiol.*, Aug 12, 52(7), 551-6.

[57] Bianchi, S., Ricci, R. P., Biscione, F., et al. (2009). Primary prevention implantation of cardioverter defibrillator without defibrillation threshold testing: 2-year follow-up. *Pacing Clin Electrophysiol.*, May, 32(5), 573-8.

[58] Michowitz, Y., Lellouche, N., Contractor, T., et al. (2011). Defibrillation threshold testing fails to show clinical benefit during long-term follow-up of patients undergoing cardiac resynchronization therapy defibrillator implantation. *Europace*, May, 13(5), 683-8.

[59] Codner, P., Nevzorov, R., & Kusniec, J. Haim. (2012). Implantable cardioverter defibrillator with and without defibrillation threshold testing. *Isr Med Assoc J.*, Jun, 14(6), 343-6.

[60] Brignole, M., Occhetta, E., Bongiorni, M. G., et al. (2012). SAFE-ICD Study Investigators. Clinical Evaluation of Defibrillation Testing in an Unselected Population of 2,120 Consecutive Patients Undergoing First Implantable Cardioverter-Defibrillator Implant. *J Am Coll Cardiol.*, Jul 24.

[61] Birnie, D., Tung, S., Simpson, D., et al. (2008). Complications Associated with Defibrillation Threshold Testing: The Canadian Experience. *Heart Rhythm*, 5, 387-390.

[62] Joglar, J. A., Kessler, D. J., Welch, P. J., et al. (1999). Effects of repeated electrical defibrillations on cardiac troponin I levels. *Am J Cardiol*, 83, 270-272, A6.

[63] Daubert, J. P., Zareba, W., & Cannom, D. S. (2008). MADIT II Investigators. Inappropriate implantable cardioverter-defibrillator shocks in MADIT II: frequency, mechanisms, predictors, and survival impact. *J Am Coll Cardiol.*, Apr 8, 51(14), 1357-65.

[64] Schwartzman, D., Callans, D. J., Gottlieb, C. D., et al. (1996). Early postoperative rise in defibrillation threshold in patients with nonthoracotomy defibrillation lead systems: Attenuation with biphasic shock waveforms. *J Cardiovasc Electrophysiol*, 7(6), 483-493.

[65] Venditti, F. J., Jr , , Martin, D. T., Vassolas, G., et al. (1994). Rise in chronic defibrillation thresholds in nonthoracotomy implantable defibrillator. *Circulation*, 89(1), 216-223.

[66] Mitchell, L. B., Pineda, E. A., Titus, J. L., et al. (2002). Sudden death in patients with implantable cardioverter defibrillators: The importance of post-shock electromechanical dissociation. *J Am Coll Cardiol*, 39(8), 1323-1328.

[67] Lever, N. A., Newall, E. G., & Larsen, P. D. (2007). Differences in the characteristics of induced and spontaneous episodes of ventricular fibrillation. *Europace*, 9, 1054-1058.

[68] Wathen, M. S., De Groot, P. J., Sweeney, M. O., et al. (2004). Prospective randomized multicenter trial of empirical antitachycardia pacing versus shocks for spontaneous rapid ventricular tachycardia in patients with implantable cardioverter-defibrillators: Pacing Fast Ventricular Tachycardia Reduces Shock Therapies (Pain-FREE Rx II) trial results. *Circulation*, 110, 2591-2596.

[69] Trappe, H. J., Wenzlaff, P., Pfitzner, P., et al. (1997). Long-term follow up of patients with implantable cardioverter-defibrillators and mild, moderate, or severe impairment of left ventricular function. *Heart*, Sep, 78(3), 243-9.

[70] Healey, J. S., Hohnloser, S. H., Glikson, M., et al. (2012). The rationale and design of the Shockless IMPLant Evaluation (SIMPLE) trial: A randomized, controlled trial of defibrillation testing at the time of defibrillator implantation. *Am Heart J.*, Aug, 164(2), 146-52.

[71] Stefano, B., Pietro, R. R., Maurizio, G., et al. (2011). Defibrillation testing during implantable cardioverter-defibrillator implantation in Italian current practice: the Assessment of Long-term Induction clinical ValuE (ALIVE) project. *Am Heart J.*, Aug, 162(2), 390-7.

Section 5

Tipps and Tricks in ICD Programming

Chapter 9

Tachycardia Discrimination Algorithms in ICDs

Martin Seifert

Additional information is available at the end of the chapter

http://dx.doi.org/10.5772/52657

1. Introduction

The detection of cardiac arrhythmia and the differential algorithm used for the recognition of ventricular tachycardia (VT) or ventricular fibrillation (VF) necessitating internal cardiac defibrillator (ICD) therapy is one of the most critical issues in ICD patients. Main goal is to develop algorithms with the highest possible sensitivity to avoid untreated arrhythmias and highest possible specificity to avoid inappropriate ICD therapies. Currently, several device discrimination algorithms and their combinations are available. The following chapter tries to explain the functionality, means, possibilities and restrictions of these ICD discrimination algorithms.

2. Cycle length / heart rate

The cycle length (CL) or heart rate (HR) is a fundament in the detection of tachycardia in ICD patients. A sustained ventricular HR in adults >250 bpm or a CL <250 ms is very specific for fast VT or VF (figure 1 red zone). However, artificial sensing of external impulses (noise), sensing caused by lead dysfunction (cluster) or inappropriate recognition of signals (T-wave-oversensing) present diagnostic challenges even in this HR zone. Below this HR almost every type of cardiac arrhythmia should be considered as well for differential diagnosis. The cycle length of both VTs and SVTs are influenced by most antiarrhythmic drugs. Therefore programming of the ICD should be accordingly adjusted.

3. VT/VF zone

In the last decade of ICD therapy the programming of a single detection zone {eg. SCD-HeFT[1]} have been replaced by the programming of up to three detection zones with different discrimination algorithms and therapies (table 1). Moreover, data on the programming of zones up to 260ms CL with a long detection time are also available {ADVANCE III study [2]}. Until now, no consensus is accepted concerning the number of detection zones (not at least in primary prevention indication), nor clear definition of detection windows is given. Until 2010 most ICDs had no SVT/VT discrimination algorithm available in the VF zone. In primary prevention a VT zone from 360ms CL with long detection time, SVT/VT discrimination up to 260ms CL and anti-tachycardia-pacing (ATP) prior or during charging, along with a VF zone from 260ms CL without SVT/VT discrimination and maximal energy shock delivery was widely recommended. Depending from device a FVT zone was needed to program an ATP prior or during charging shock up to 280-250ms CL. Newer devices have now independent discrimination algorithm for every detection zone (Medtronic), and provide SVT/VT discrimination algorithms also in VF zone. Furthermore, ATPprior or during charging is available in all zones. In secondary prevention patients with documented VTs, the first zone should be programmed 10-20ms above (or 10 bpm below) its cycle length. In younger patients with channel rhythm disorders like long QT syndrome a single zone (<280ms) can be considered. Patients with secondary prevention, very low ejection fraction or repetitive syncope need an individualized, more conservative programming with shorter detection intervals and less ATPs. Different programming examples for tachycardia detection and therapies in recent studies with primary prevention patients with ICDs of different manufacturers are listed in table 1.

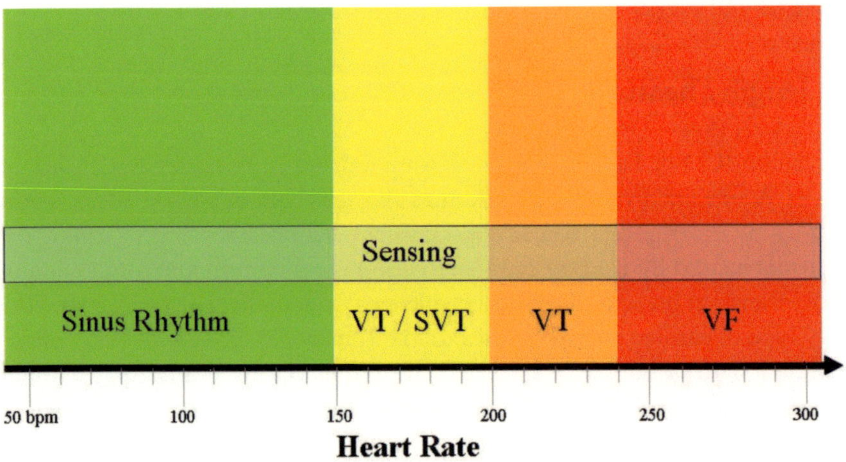

Figure 1. Notice critical area of VT and VF discrimination in yellow and orange up to 460ms cycle length

Practically, devices in primary prevention patients can be programmed using either single or two zones with long detection intervals. The programming should be adjusted during the follow-up in case of arrhythmic events.

zone	VT	FVT	VF
Study, date and manufactures	**150bpm**	**200bpm**	**250bpm**
SCD-HeFT[1] 2005 Medtronic		187bpm [18/24 beats) only Shocks	
PAINFREE[13] I 2001 Medtronic	Rx – 188 bpm[12/16] ATPx2 → Shocks	188 – 250 bpm[12/16 beats) ATPx2 → Shocks	>250 bpm[12/16 beats) Shocks only
PAINFREE[14] II 2005 Medtronic	167 – 188 bpm[18/24] ATPx3 → Shocks	188 – 250 bpm[18/24 beats) ATPx1 → Shocks vs Shocks only	>250 bpm[18/24 beats) Shocks only
EMPIRIC[15] 2006 Medtronic	150 – 200 bpm[16 beats) ATPx3 → Shocks	200 – 250 bpm[18/24 beats) ATPx1 → Shocks	>250 bpm[18/24 beats) Shocks only
PREPARE[16] 2008 Medtronic	167 – 182 bpm [32 beats) Monitor	182 – 250 bpm[30/40 beats) ATPx1 → Shocks	>250 bpm[30/40 beats) Shocks only
ADVANCE III[2] Medtronic 2012		187bpm [30/40 beats) ATP during change	
MADIT[17] 1996 Boston	no clear definition	no clear definition	
MADIT II[6] 2002 Boston	170 – 200 bpm, [1-5 sec delay) discrimination free, therapy free or Monitor	>200 bpm[1-3 sec delay) Shocks	
MADIT CRT[18] 2011 Boston Scientific	170 – 200 bpm [60s delay), Rhythm ID ATPx1 → Shocks	200 – 250 bpm [12 sec delay) Rhythm ID ATPx1 → Shocks	>250 bpm[2.5 sec delay) Quick Convert ATP → Shocks
PROVIDE St.Jude Medical ongoing 2008-"/> (NCT00743522]	181 – 214 bpm [25 beats) SVT Discr. ATPx2 → Shocks	214 – 250 bpm[18 beats) ATPx1 → Shocks	>250bpm [12 beats) Shocks only

Table 1. Change in detection for defibrillation therapy over the last ten years in corner stone studies of different manufactures.

4. Inappropriate ICD therapy

Inappropriate ICD therapy is a delivered ATP and/or shock in absence of VT/VF episode. Inappropriate ICD therapy has serious consequences: proarrhythmic effect, reduced quality of life, psychological stress with depression, unnecessary hospitalisation, early battery depletion duration and even elevated mortality [3]. Up to 80% of inappropriate ICD therapies are registered in the first year following device implantation [4, 5] figure 2. Atrial fibrillation

(AF) is the most common cause of inappropriate ICD therapy {MADIT II [6], figure 3}. However, concerning the rising number of lead dysfunction resulting in oversensing this can be changed in the future. In the SCD-HeFT[3] study with single zone of detection and therapy (18 of 24 beats at a rate ≥188 bpm or ≤320 ms CL) the effect of inappropriate versus appropriate ICD therapy to the hazard ratio for death (CI 95%) was 1.98 (p=0.002) for inappropriate therapy only (figure 4).It is unclear whether the inappropriate therapy is a cause or only a marker of higher mortality. By all means, consensus exists about the importance of avoiding inappropriate ICD therapies. The incidence of inappropriate ICD therapy depends on the programming of the device – both detection and therapy, and considerable changes were observed over the last years (table 2).

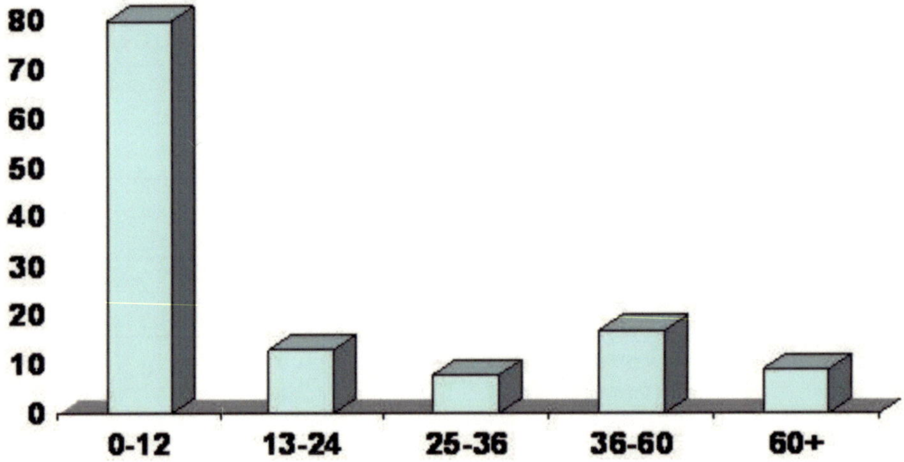

Figure 2. Frequency (y line in %) of inappropriate ICD therapies after ICD implantation (x line in month, y line in %) Nanthakumar K et al[5].

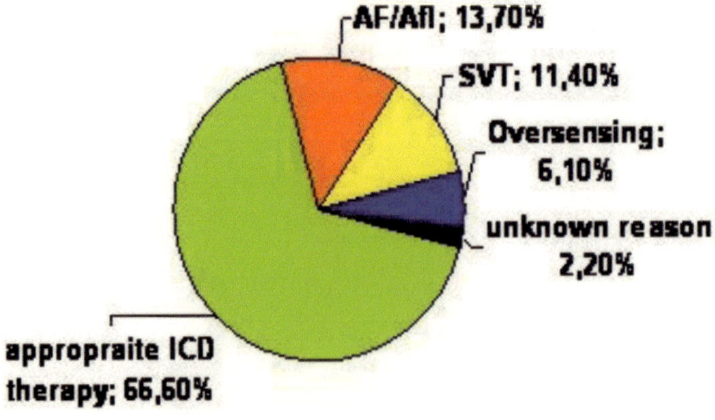

Figure 3. Reasons of inappropriate ICD therapy in MADIT II [4].

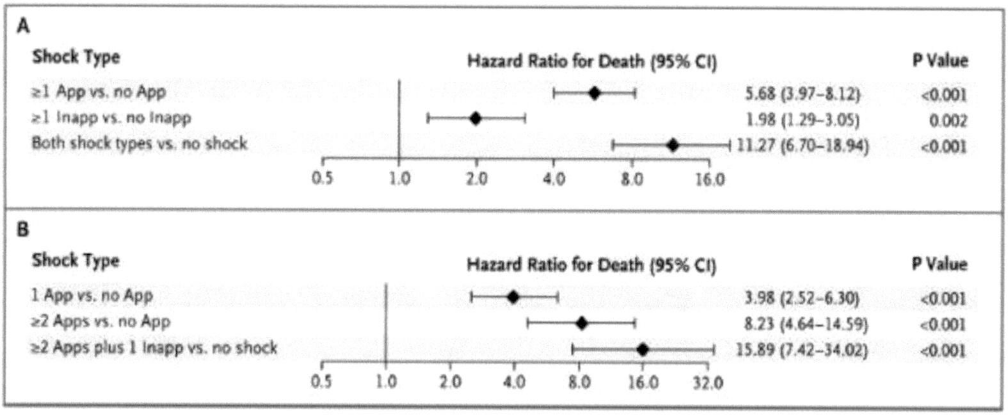

Figure 4. Relation of appropriate and inappropriate ICD therapy in SCD-HeFT to mortality [3].

Year	Author	Mean age	Patients (n)	% appropriate ICD therapy	% inappropriate ICD therapy
1996	Weber et al[19]		462	55	18
2002	Daubert et al[4]	63	719	66	11,5
2003	Nanthakumar et al[5]	60	261	54	44
2004	Rinald et al[20]	60	155		14
2007	Anselmeet al[21]	64	802	28	15
2008	Wilkoff et al[16]	67	700	5,4 (shock, not ATP)	3,6 (shock, not ATP)

Table 2. Incidences of appropriate and inappropriate ICD therapies over the last years. Notice the influence of SVT/VT discrimination algorithm until CL of 260ms and longer detection intervals.

5. Detection Time (DT) or Number of Interval Detection (NID)

Detection of tachycardia occurs after the registration of a certain amount of heartbeats within or above the programmed HR zone. Signals with CL according to VF zone have priority to signals in VT zone(s). Various algorithms are currently used for validation of a tachycardia: registering of a specified and programmed number of beats - x out of y (Medtronic and Biotronik, figure 5), a programmed number of beats (x) with resetting after 5 consecutive below-zonebeats (St. Jude Medical, figure 6) or after a programmed time interval (Boston, figure 7). During the last years programming of a long detection time has been established in primary prophylactic indication (figure 8 and table 1).

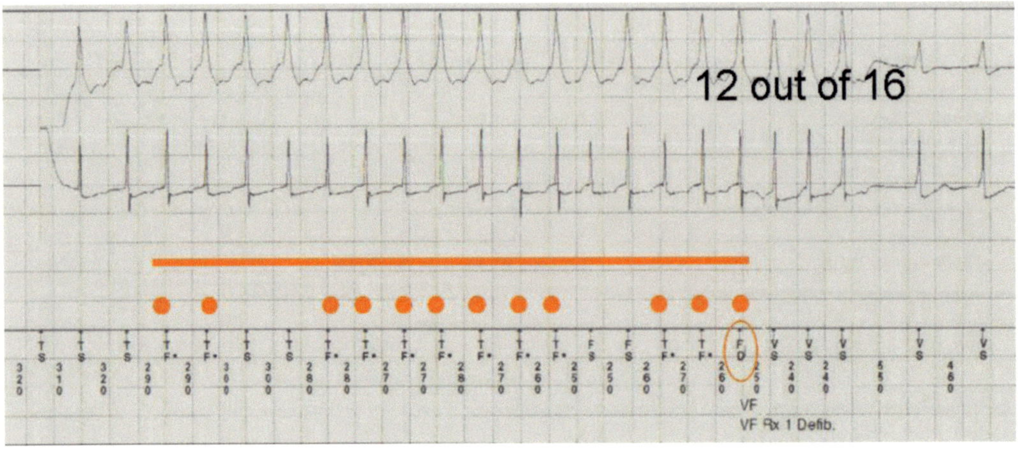

Figure 5. Tachycardia detection of a Medtronic device: TS tachycardia sense in VT1 zone; VS ventricular sense; TF fibrillation sense via VT2 zone; FS fibrillation sense. In this case x=12 (<300ms orange points) out of y=16 signals counted for detection of a VF episode with spontaneous conversion to sinus rhythm after 22 beats.

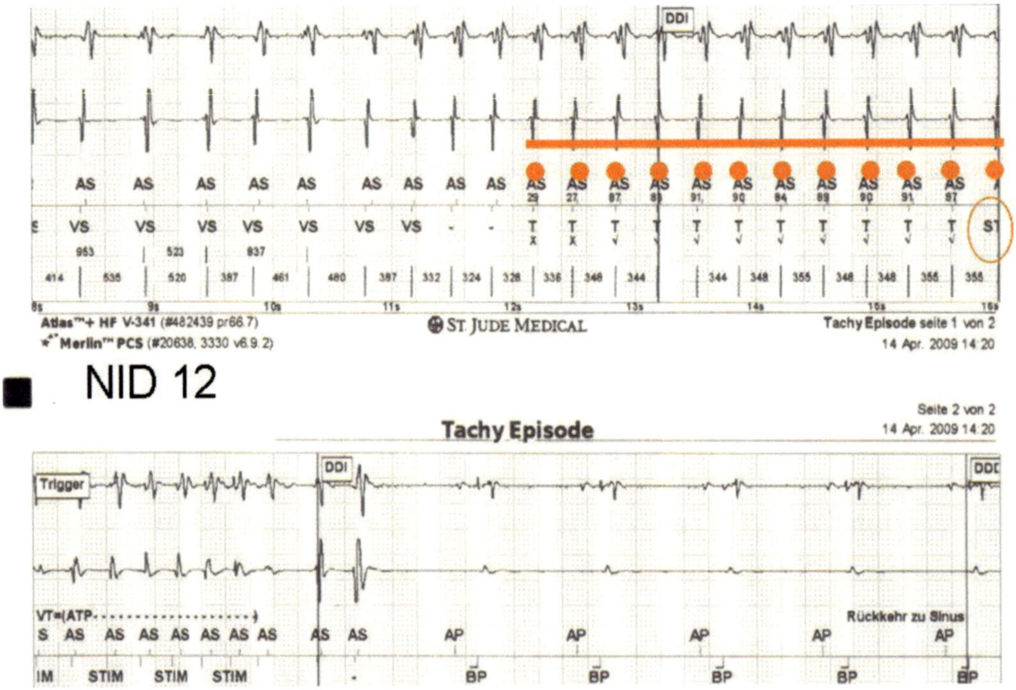

Figure 6. Tachycardia detection of a CRT device from St. Jude Medical (dual chamber detection): VS ventricle sense; AS atrial sense; T tachycardia sense in VT zone; ST tachycardia episode sense; X no correspondence with stored QRS templet; little minced meat correspondence with stored templet, NID x=12 (orange points) counted to VT episode with successful ATP. The episode shows a short VA interval with accelerated CL and corresponding templet to intrinsic activation. That means episode could diagnose as VT with VA conduction and wrong stored templet or as SVT (atrioventricular node reentry tachycardia) with atypical start.

http://dx.doi.org/10.5772/52657

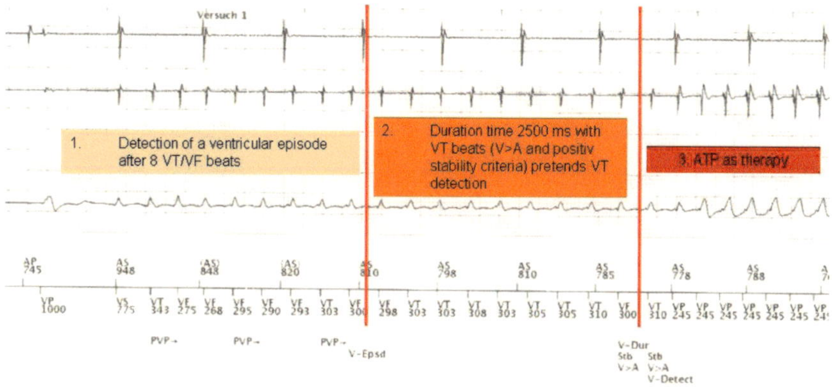

Figure 7. Tachcardia detection of a dual chamber device Boston: VS ventricle sense; AS atrial sense (AS) refracted; PVP atrial refracted after ventricle sense; VT ventricular tachycardia sense; VF ventricular fibrillation in VF zone sense; V-Epsd ventricular episode ready for duration; V-Dur duration time complete; Stb stability criteria is right; V-Detect ventricular episodes is detected and therapy ATP begins.

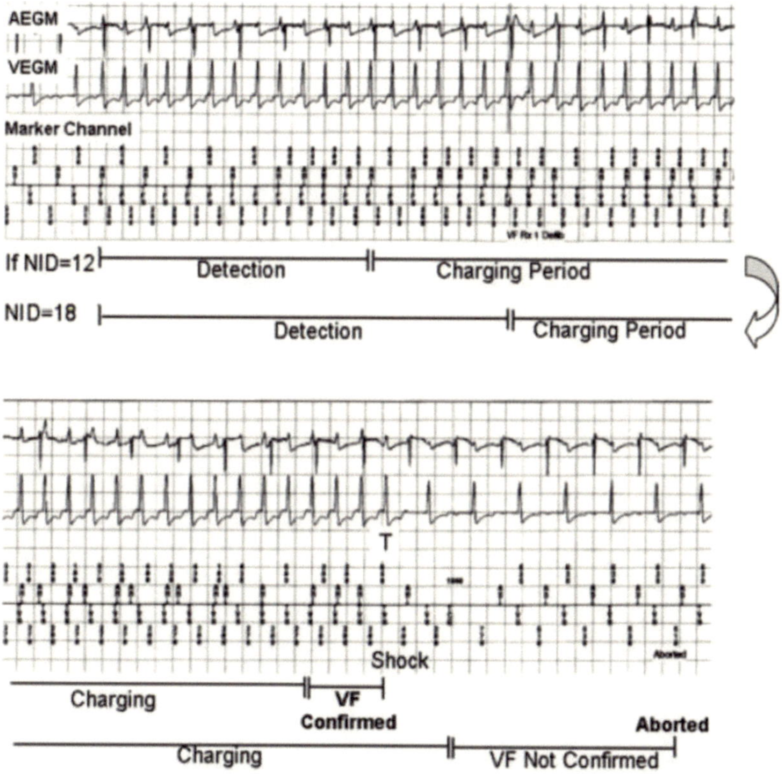

Figure 8. Gunderson at al [23] demonstrate ICD shock therapy which is delivered or aborted in the same VT episode according to detection interval NID 12 or 18.

6. Discrimination SVT/VT

Discrimination of SVT and VT may present a challenge not only for devices using artificial intelligence and programmed algorithms but even for experienced physicians. Principally the following wide QRS complex arrhythmias should be considered: VT, SVT with bundle branch block, SVT with accessory pathway or pacing in left (via coronary sinus) or right ventricle. Table 3 shows the discrimination criteria of the 12 channel ECG for SVT/VT. No single criterion is sensitive and specific enough to provide sufficient discrimination value. Therefore, combination of several criteria should be implemented in the device algorithms to correctly diagnose arrhythmias. Table 4 shows the availability of discrimination criteria in single or dual chamber ICDs.

ECG criteria	sensitivity	specificity
QRS width	high	low
VA dissociation	low	high
capture beats	low	high
northwest axis	low	high
rS missed or long rS in V1	low	medium
concordance +/-	low	high
Brugada criteria LBBB/RBBB[22]	medium	high

Table 3. Sensitivity (in sense of frequency) and specificity of different ECG criteria for differentiation SVT and VT.

criteria	ECG	Single chamber	Dual chamber
CL or heart rate	+	+	+
stability	+	+	+
Sudden onset	+ (Holter ECG)	+	+
morphology	+	+	+
AV rate branch	-	-	+
QRS axis (*Rhythm ID™ Boston)	+	+(*)	+(*)
AVA interval	-	-	+
Sinus Interval History (*St. Jude Medical)	-	+(*)	-
Capture beats (*PR Logic™Medtronic)	+	-	+(*)
RBBB and LBBB criterias	+	-	-

Table 4. Variation of SVT and VT discrimination criteria in single and dual chamber ICDs (+ achievable; - not achievable).

7. Stability

Stability is the variability of tachycardia CL (figure 9). In general, VTs have a reasonably stable CL while numerous SVTs have beat-to-beat variability in their CL (AF, Sinus tachycardia, etc). However, some SVTs may have stable CL as well: circus movement tachycardia, atrioventricular nodal re-entry tachycardia or atrial flutter (Aflut) – so this criterion has his limitations. Even AF may have a quite stable CL in the case of very high frequency. Anyway, several randomized controlled studies {e.g. MADIT II [7]} proved a significant decrease (p=0.030) of inappropriate ICD therapies (table 5). Therefore, programming of stability criterion is recommended in single chamber devices up to 260ms CL and indual chamber devices in the case V <A. The programmed value depends on the manufacturer, and lies in general for single and dual chamber devices around 40ms (-20 to + 20ms) [8]. Boston and St. Jude Medical use the last 12 consecutive intervals and compare the second longest and the shortest interval to calculate the difference in ms (or percentage ratio). Medtronic and Biotronik use the last 3 and 4 consecutive intervals to calculate mean difference.

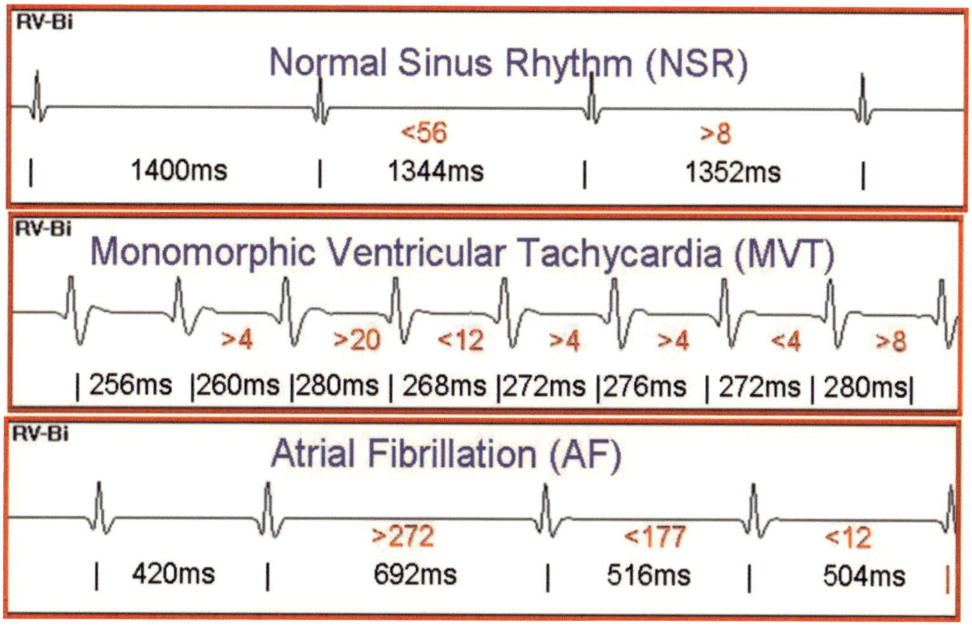

Figure 9. Notice variability of CL in ms (in red numbers) from beat to beat in normal sinus rhythm, monomorphic ventricular tachycardia and atrial fibrillation AF.

8. Sudden onset

Initiation of the tachycardia may also provide information on the mechanism and origin of the arrhythmia. The heart rate in the case of a sinus tachycardia at physical activity rises slowly and gradually. Other SVTs or ventricular arrhythmias cause a sudden and marked jump in the heart rate (or fall in CL). Primary role of the Sudden onset criterion is therefore the diagnose of sinus tachycardia (figures 10 and 11). However, in some studies the algorithm using this criterion resulted in delayed VT detection (figure 12) or could not show significant reduction of inappropriate ICD therapy (table 5). Therefore, programming of sudden onset criterion is recommended above all in younger patients who could reach high HR at physical activity and could tolerate longer the hemodynamic consequences of a potential VT. This group is generally underrepresented in large ICD studies, which may be the reason why the effect on the incidence of inappropriate ICD therapy could not be proven.

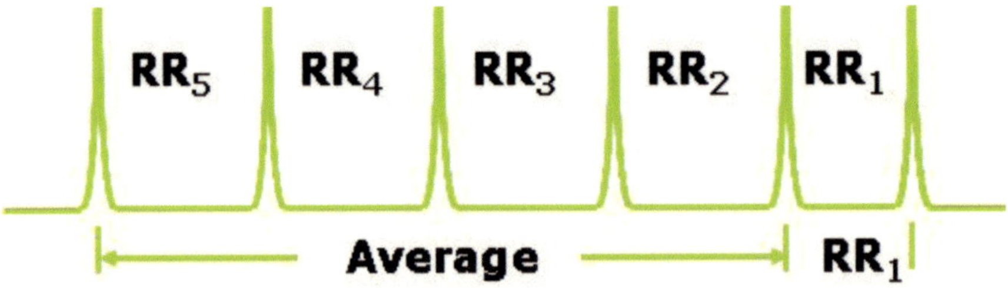

Figure 10. Demonstration of sudden onset calculation: The device compares RR1 with mean from RR2 to RR5 (Biotronik), onset (%) = (RR1*100]/mean from RR2 to RR5 for Boston, standard 10% or for Medtronic graduated onset (%) mean from RR1 to RR4 / mean RR5 to RR8, standard 81%

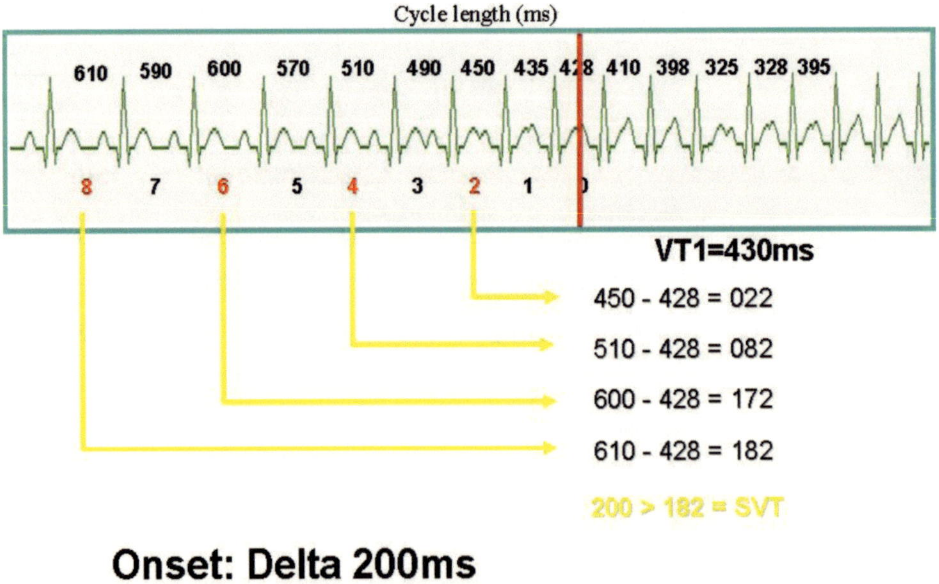

Figure 11. Demonstration of the St. Jude Medical algorithm for sudden onset (standard Δ150-160]. In this case of Δ <200ms the algorithm decides for SVT.

Programming	Inappropriate shock	No inappropriate shock	P value
Single chamber			
Number of patients	83	83	
Lowest VT zone (beats/min)	169.3 ± 19.9	171.9 ± 14.5	0.540
Lowest VT zone detection time (s)	2.45 ± 1.99	2.42 ± 2.07	0.830
Stability on % (n)	17 (14)	36 (30)	0.030
Sudden onset on % (n)	16 (13	23 (19)	0.160
Dual chamber			
Number of patients	32	36	
V>a on% (n)	31 (10)	50 (18)	0.054
Atrial fibrillation discriminator on % (n)	34 (11)	44 (16)	0.210

Table 5. Influences of discrimination algorithms to inappropriate ICD-shock according to single and dual chamber detection in MADIT II trial [4].

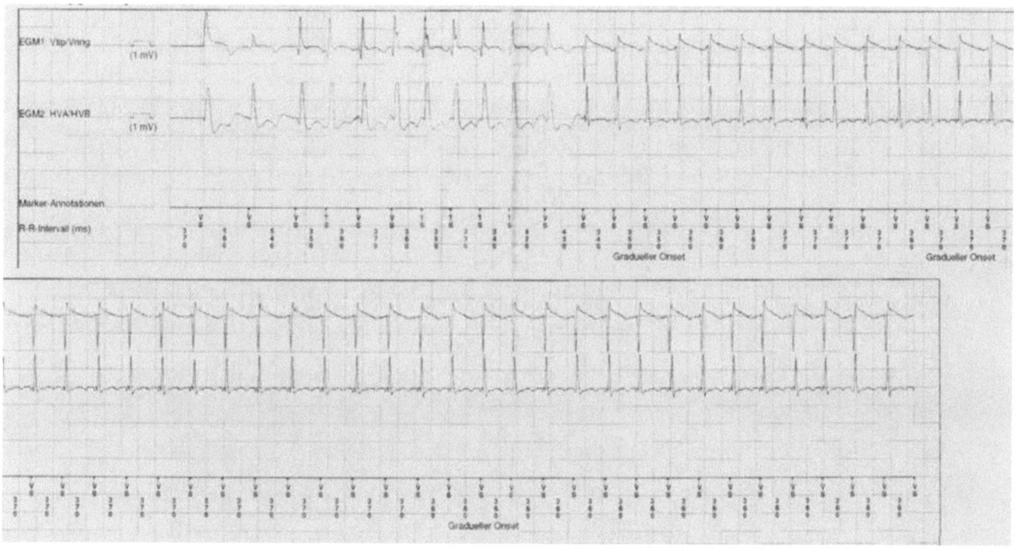

Figure 12. Notice prolonged detection of sustained VT caused by graduated onset algorithm of a Medtronic device. There is a VT with obviously change in vector and stable CL of 370 ms. The graduated onset is calculated graduated caused by 10 beats of another tachycardia leads to a negative sudden onset criteria.

9. Timer

Depending from manufacturers a time window can be defined for SVT/VT discrimination in VT zones. In case of an episode identified as SVT the device may suspend the programmed therapy only within this specified time interval, when the time runs out, the device delivers VT therapy (SVT time out). Also in case of an episode identified as VT the device may switch to the VF therapy after a specified time interval (VT time out). Generally these counters are not recommended because SVTs usually continue for longer time periods and such timer could force an ATP or shock delivery inappropriately. However, in individual cases (e.g. in patients with very low ejection fraction who could not tolerate higher HR for a longer time) programming a time out intervals may be considered for safety reasons.

10. Morphology criteria

Morphology and width of QRS complexes is a primary tool for physicians to differentiate SVT from VT (table 3 and 4). Accordingly, almost all manufacturers have developed QRS complex morphology algorithms. The device compare 8 or more voltage points on the EGM signals at different time points (figure 13). A point to point assessment of each complex to a defined standard complex (template) follows. Finally, decision is made based on a previously programmed matching-ratio in percentage (figure 14). Currently, programming of this criterion is recommended in single chamber devices and in dual chamber devices in case of V<A and V=A. The algorithms use either EGM only or a combination of EGM and a can to coil lead (figure 15). In case of no intrinsic activation like third degree atrioventricular block or continuous biventricular pacing the automatic storing algorithm of QRS complex template may be problematic or even not possible. In the latter case QRS template should be stored manually during pacing inhibition. In case of HR dependent bundle branch block this algorithm may also fail to differentiate tachycardias.

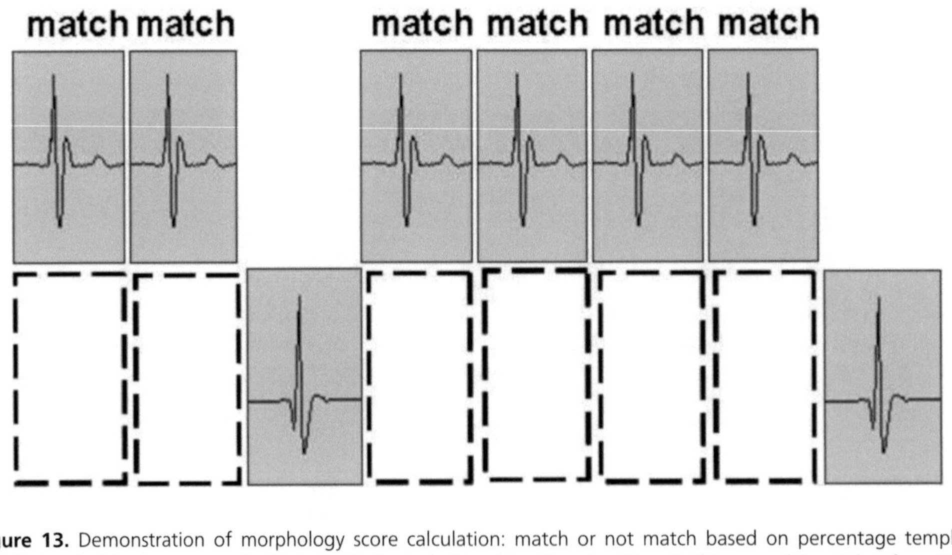

Figure 13. Demonstration of morphology score calculation: match or not match based on percentage template match threshold measurement by St. Jude Medical window detection algorithm. In this case of 6 matches from 8 the algorithm votes for SVT [75%).

http://dx.doi.org/10.5772/52657

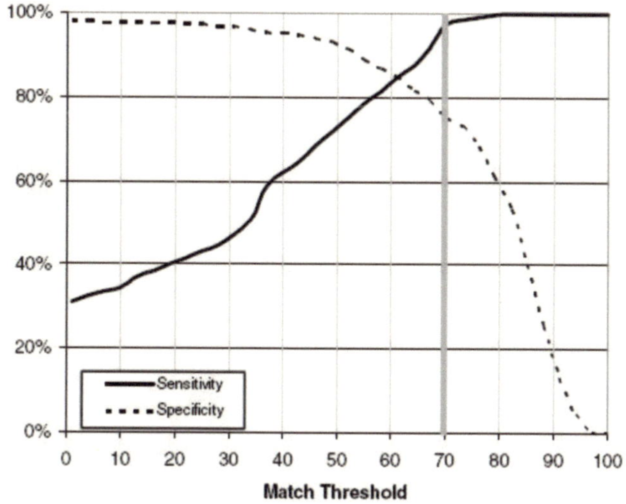

Figure 14. Demonstration of sensitivity and specify of the Medtronic Wavelet™ algorithm to differentiate between SVT and VT by Klein et al [24]. As recommendation a value of 70% match is standard by Medtronic devices.

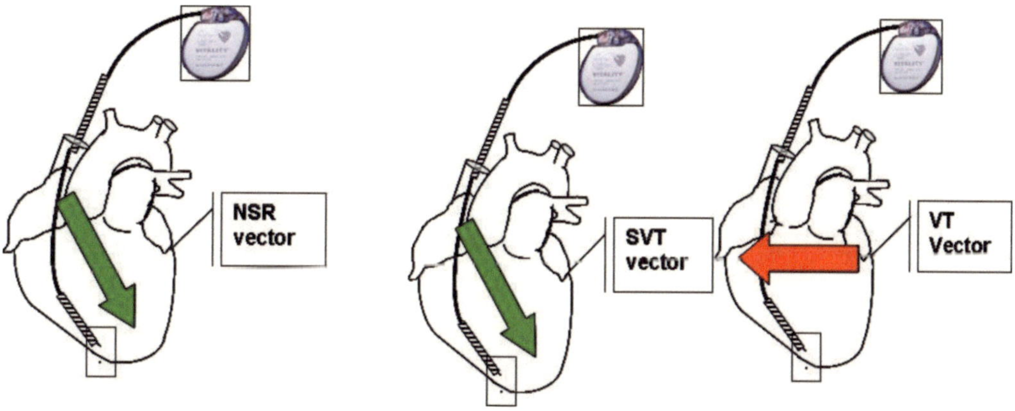

Figure 15. Demonstration of the Rhythm ID™ discrimination algorithm: discrimination between sinus rhythm and SVT with "normal" vector (green) to a potential VT vector (red). This algorithm is not based on EGM signal but on an internal ECG electrode from device can to RV shock coil and the vena cava shock coil.

11. SVT/VT discrimination algorithms in single chamber devices

In the programming of single chamber ICD the three most important discrimination criteria are stability, morphology and sudden onset. However, it should be defined whether a single criterion or only matching of all three criteria should rule out a VT. Currently, if all three criteria are active, it is recommended to rule out VT in case of 2 out of 3 votes for SVT. If only two criteria are active (standard), stability and morphology are recommended, and 1 out 2 votes is required for the diagnosis of SVT. Anyway, differentiation between SVT and VT in single as well as dual chamber ICD remains difficult and should be carefully checked by the physician at each follow-up visit (figure 16a-b).

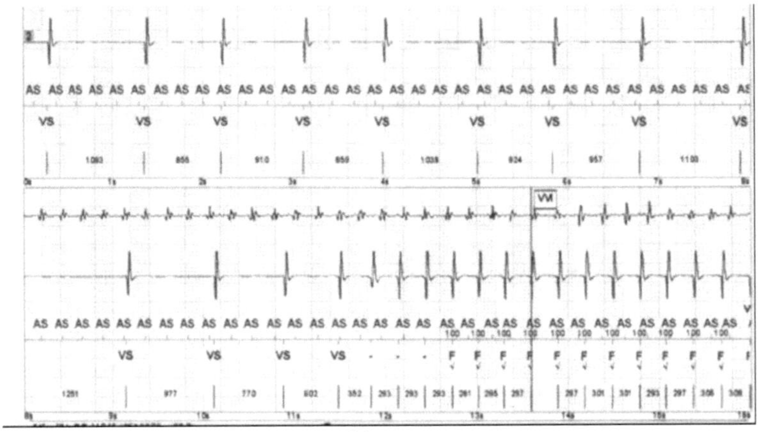

(a)

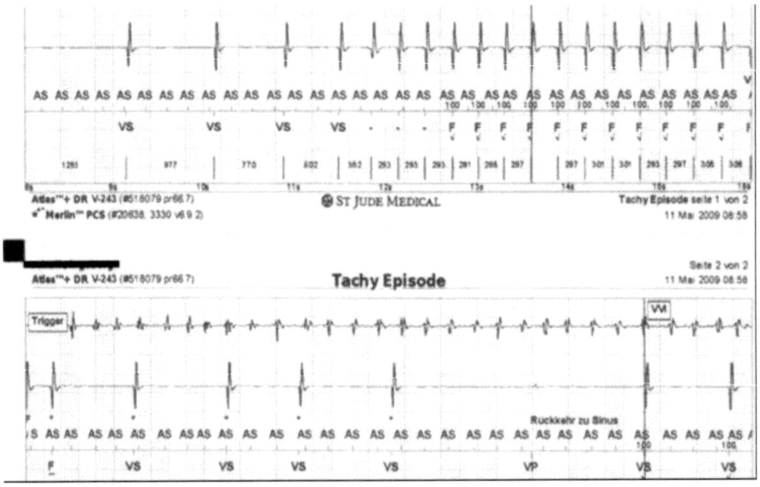

(b)

Figure 16. a: This episode of a dual chamber tachycardia detection (Atlas DR St. Jude Medical) with A>V during AF with a CL around 100ms demonstrates the hardly difficult decision-making in spite of all common discrimination algorithms. The ventricular EGM shows a fast stable tachycardia with a CL of around 300ms and sudden onset as well as nearly same EGM signal like intrinsic activation before. This tachycardia falls in VF zone and the morphology criteria founds a match to intrinsic activation of stored template. Although morphology votes for SVT, stability outvote for VT <40ms (sudden onset not active), but anyway the CL falls in VF zone in this case without active SVT discrimination algorithm the device detected this episode as VF and start charging shock therapy (*). b: The same episode stopped spontaneously without any therapy and the shock is aborted by the device. The example underlined the importance of long detection intervals (TDI 18-24 not 12 like in this case), the need of competent discrimination algorithm also in short CL under 300ms and the difficult interpretation of an episode not only by the device but also by physicians in decision making SVT or VT.

12. SVT/VT discrimination algorithms in dual chamber devices

Detection and diagnose of arrhythmias in dual chamber devices is more complex, and the mechanism of decision making is harder to demonstrate. Discrimination algorithms are still based on the principles explained above. Significant addition is the comparison of atrial (A) and ventricular (V) frequency (figure 17). In case of V>A VT therapy is initiated directly. For cases with V=A or V<A further discrimination algorithms are used to differentiate between SVT and VT. For V<A programming of morphology and stability criteria is recommended. For V=A programming of morphology criterion may be sufficient. In addition for V<A episodes measurement of the A-V-A intervals may differentiate SVTs with 2:1 activation from VTs with VA dissociation during AF/Aflut. Measurement of A-V-A intervals by St. Jude Medical devices (AV Detection Enhance™) is illustrated in figure 18a-b. This algorithm counts the last 12 AV intervals and calculates the difference between the second longest and second shortest AV interval; difference < 40ms suggests association between A and V and decides for SVT. A comparable algorithm based on pattern recognition typical for Aflut or SVT with 1:1 AV-conduction is used by Medtronic called PR-Logic™ and by Biotronik called SMART™. Sorin use an algorithm more orientated to CL stability called PARAD(+)™[9].

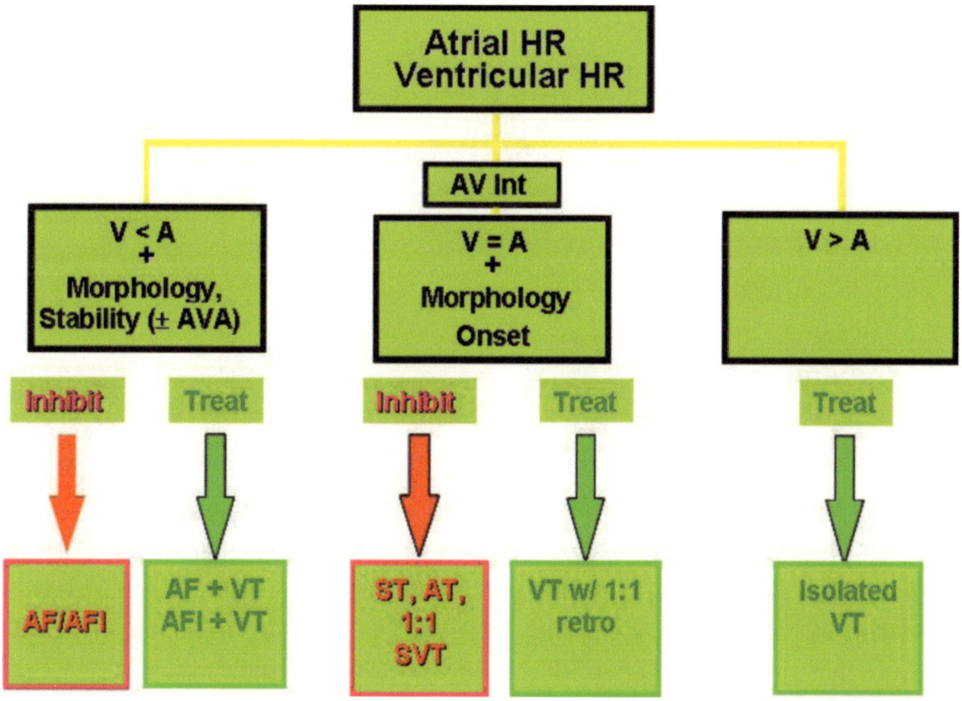

Figure 17. The rate branch differentiates between V<A, V=A and V>A. For VA dissociation a VT will therapies by ICD directly. In case of V=A a sinus tachycardia or other 1:1 SVT should inhibited by ICD and in case of retrograde activation of a VT the ICD should delivered therapy. For V<A and AF/AFl therapy should inhibited and V<A with VT and current AF/AFl therapy should delivered.

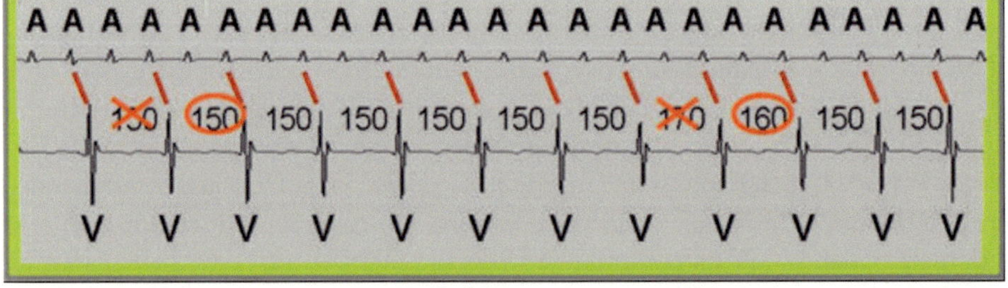

(a)

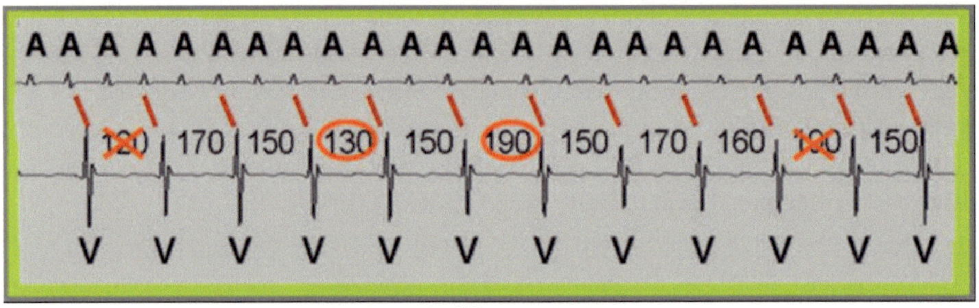

(b)

Figure 18. a: This is an example for measurement AV association during AFl with 2:1 activation. Although stability says stable CL <40ms there is an association between A and V. 160-150ms = 10ms for AVA interval (standard < 40ms for SVT) indicate association with RA. The algorithm vote for SVT and AVA interval outvotes stability. b: This is an example for measurement AV dissociation during AFl and VT. The second longest minus second shortest AV interval (190ms-130ms=60ms) is voted by delta >40ms for dissociation and VT.

13. Tachy/Sinus ratio

Tachy/Sinus ratio counter is an algorithm from St. Jude Medical to avoid oversensing bigeminy during sinus tachycardia, t-wave oversensing or cluster caused by lead fracture. In figure 19 calculation of CL ratio of 2.5 (500ms/200ms) over the last 12 sinus beats is illustrated. For every ratio of 2.5 the algorithm counts -1, and for counter <3 over the last 12 beats the algorithm votes for bigeminy and for >3 for VT. Medtronic has developed an algorithm called Lead Integrity Alert™; a short RR counter combined with daily lead impedance monitoring as early warning system for lead fracture. These algorithms have growing importance due to the rising number of lead fracture problems over the last years. Biotronik also developed its t-wave detection protection algorithm. Furthermore, all manufacturers use an automatic gain control as dynamic sense control to avoid t-wave oversensing.

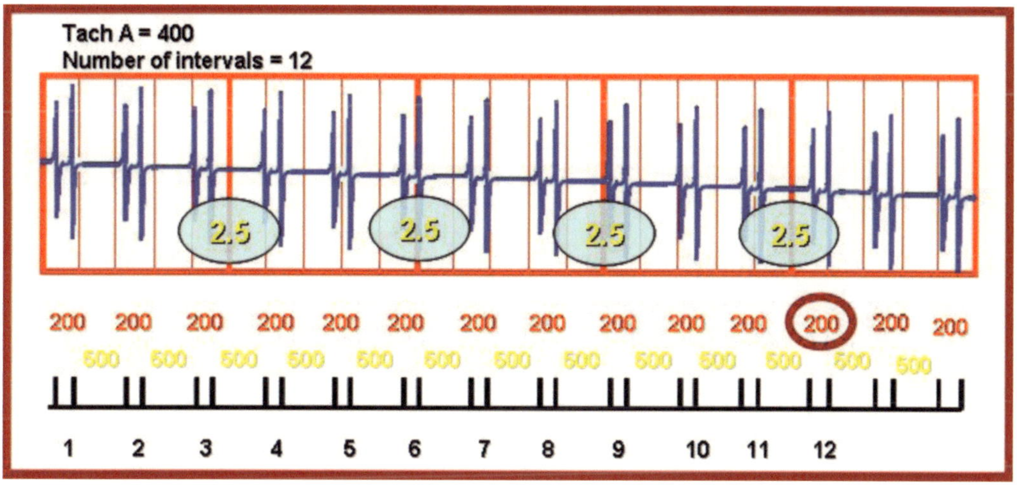

Figure 19. This is an example for measurement Tachy/Sinus ratio. Over the last 12 interval the ratio 500/200 turns out 2.5. For this value the algorithm counts -1 and calculate this over the last 12 beats. For a value <3 SVT and >3 VT is assumed.

14. Decision making for single or dual chamber ICD

In the last decade the issue of implanting single or dual chamber ICD was thoroughly discussed. The negative influence of ventricular pacing in DAVID I trial [10] could be avoided in the DAVID II trial [11], which demonstrated similar prognoses in single and dual chamber patients for freedom of unfavourable ventricular pacing. The 1&1 trail of Bansch et al [9] failed (p=0.08) to demonstrate superiority of dual chamber devices to prevent inappropriate therapy in ICD patients. Also in MADIT II no benefit for dual chamber ICD patients could be confirmed [4]. The Detect SVT study by Friedman et al [12] could show a significant decrease of inappropriate therapy in dual chamber patients (with 30.9% in 1,090 episodes versus 39.5% in 1,253 episodes in single chamber ICD patients (p=0,03, see figure 20). Superiority was reported in the diagnose of AF, Aflut and atrial tachycardia (figure 21). No benefit could be demonstrated in sinus tachycardia, lead dysfunction and t-wave oversensing. Still, even dual chamber ICDs may fail to discriminate appropriately (figure 22a-f). This figure also may help to explain why inappropriate ICD therapy could have a negative effect on mortality in ICD patients. An recently, not jet published abstract of HRS congress 2012 of Friedman et al. of a prospective randomized trail of dual chamber versus single chamber ICD to minimize shocks in optimally programmed devices with optimal 30/40 detection of Medtronic devices no significant superiority of dual chamber devices could measure in attention to inappropriate therapies. Significant more AF was detected in the dual chamber device group. Generally, the choice of single or dual chamber does not depend on the intention of a better SVT discrimination (e.g. patients with paroxysmal AF). Main indication for dual chamber ICD is the necessity of atrial pacing.

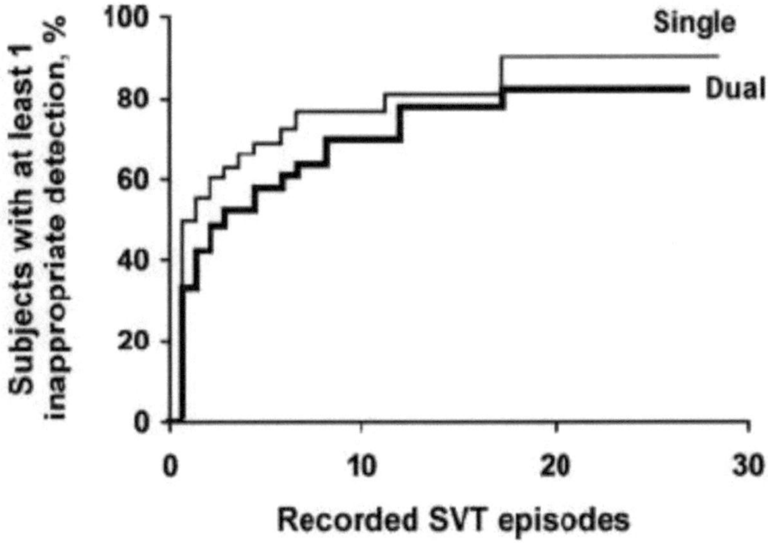

Figure 20. Comparison of inappropriate SVT detection in single and dual chamber ICDs. Notice 30.9% inappropriate SVT detection in 1,090 episodes in dual chamber versus 39.5% in 1,253 episodes in single chamber ICD patients (p=0.03) [12].

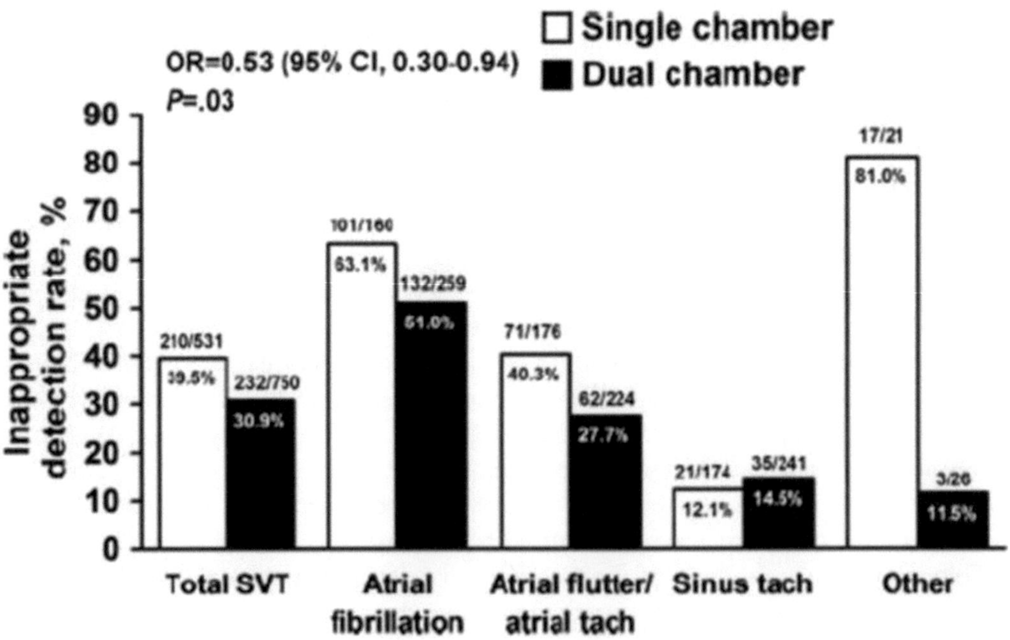

Figure 21. Comparison of inappropriate SVT detection in single and dual chamber ICDs. A trend for superiority was estimated in AF, AFl and atrial tachycardia in the Detect SVT study [12].

http://dx.doi.org/10.5772/52657

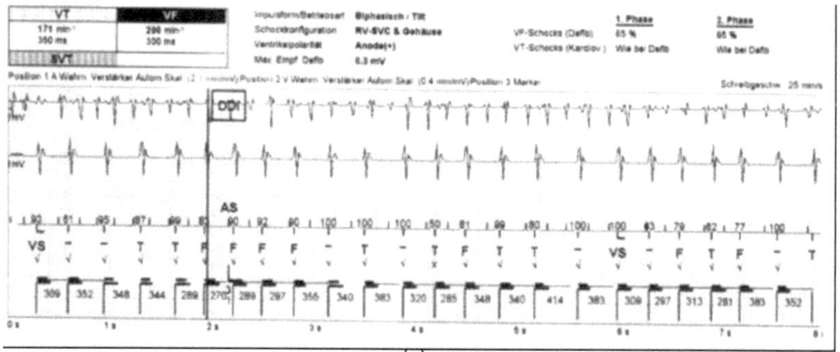

(a)

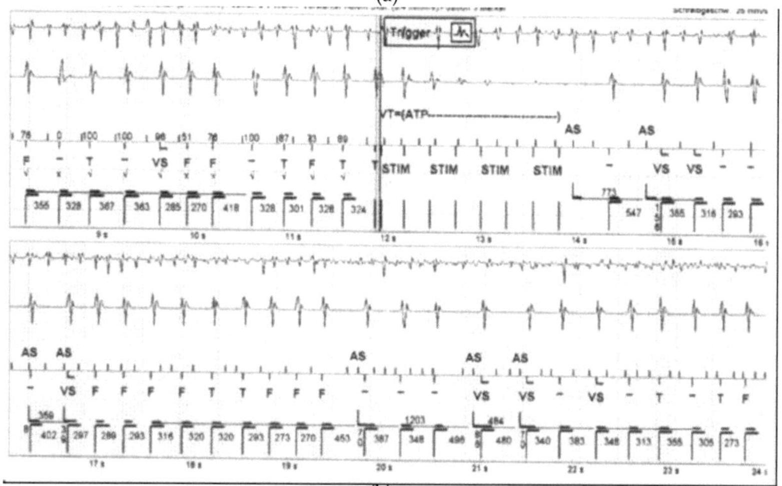

(b)

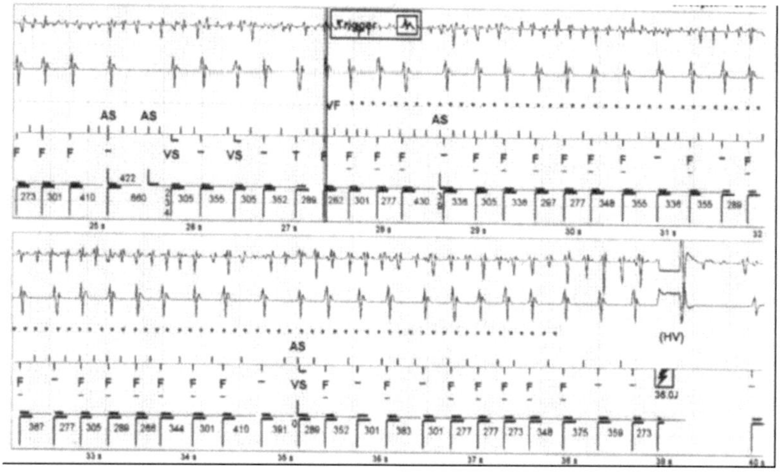

(c)

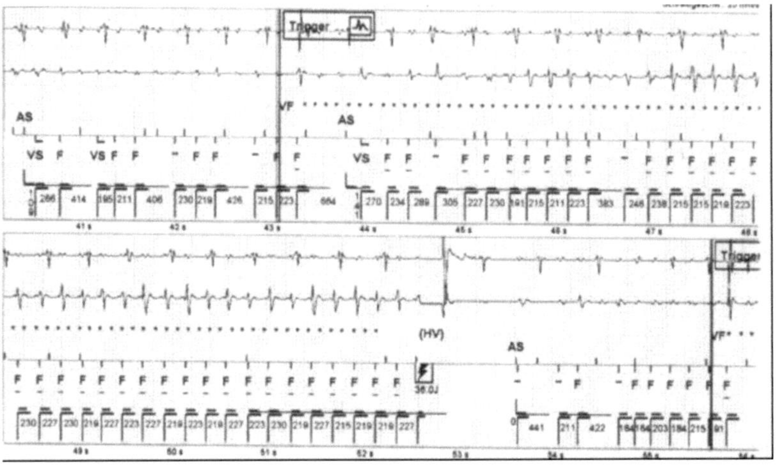

(d)

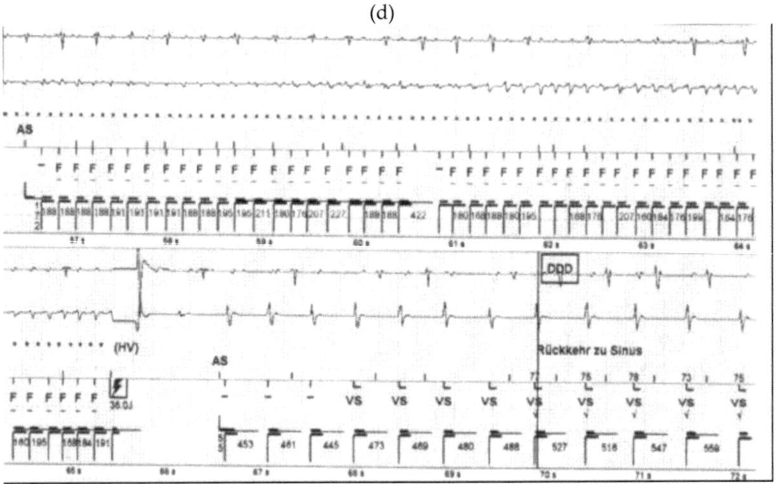

(e)

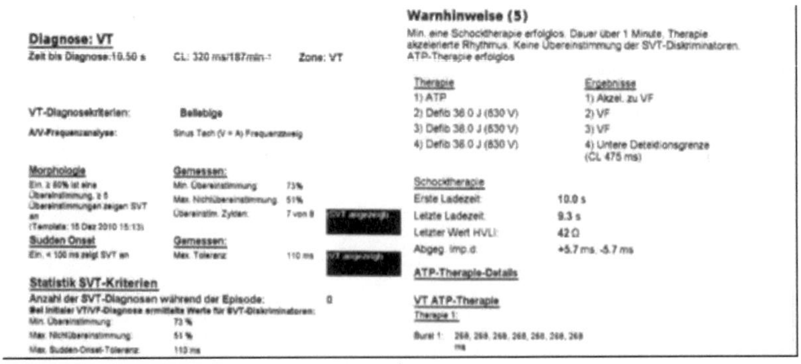

(f)

Figure 22. a: Demonstration of an AF episode in a CRT-D device with dual chamber detection (Promote St. Jude Medical) A>V with CL around 344 to 270ms. Depending of CL the device counts VT (T) and VF (F) beats for detection. In this device no SVT discrimination algorithms are allowed in VF zone. b: Same episode 12 seconds later. After detection VT episode (NID 12] first VT therapy (ATP) is given. c: Same episode 27 seconds later. After acceleration of AF a VF episode

http://dx.doi.org/10.5772/52657

is detected (NID 12] and the first shock is delivered. d: Same episode 43 seconds later. After the first shock ventricular fibrillation with syncope of patient is following, second shock (ineffective) at second 52 of episode is delivered. e: Same episode 65 seconds later. The third shock, now effective, is delivered during ventricular fibrillation and episode ends with sinus rhythm.f: This picture of the same episode turns out reasons for detection of AF in the VT zone. A temporary AF undersensing in RA rolls this episode in V=A branch. Generally based from 1:1 tachycardia in this branch stability is not sensible and programmed in this branch. In this case there are morphology and sudden onset discrimination active. For understandable reasons morphology votes for SVT and sudden onset for VT and resulting VT therapy starts. As previously described sudden onset criteria is not recommended in this branch and an always problematic discrimination algorithm.

15. Summary/Conclusion

Avoiding of inappropriate therapy delivery is one of the major issues in ICD therapy. In the last decade several new algorithms were developed to improve sensitivity and specificity of tachycardia detection. Current recommendation for primary prevention patients is the programming of a fast VT zone from 187 to 250 bpm with long NID or DT [30/40] for Medtronic, 12 seconds for Boston, 18/24 for St. Jude Medical and Biotronik), is ATP prior or during charging followed by shock therapy. For devices that not allow SVT discrimination in this zone a separate VF zone above 250 bpm should be programmed to make SVT discrimination possible in a VT zone of 187 to 250 bpm. If a second VT zone around 150-187 bpm is programmed, a long NID (minimum 25 beats or 60 seconds) with stability and morphology discrimination algorithm without time out rule is recommended. Algorithms for early detection of lead fracture, sinus/tachy ratio and impedance monitoring are recommended when available. In patients with long QT syndrome or other risk for primary VF a single zone over 220 bpm is recommended. In dual chamber ICDs stability, morphology and A-V-A (or equivalent) SVT discrimination algorithms are recommended in the analysis of V=A and V<A tachycardias. Implantation of dual chamber ICD for better SVT/VT discrimination only is not indicated by currently available studies.

No algorithm is sensitive or specific enough to substitute the individual adaptation of ICD detection and therapy for every patient. Detailed knowledge of ICD algorithms may provide the necessary basis for the cardiologist to program devices individualized for each patient. Stored episodes should be carefully evaluated at every follow-up visit to further improve discrimination of SVTs and VTs.

Author details

Martin Seifert*

Address all correspondence to: m.seifert@immanuel.de

Heartcenter Brandenburg and Immanuel Klinikum Bernau, Department of Cardiology, Bernau bei Berlin, Germany

References

[1] Bardy GH, Lee KL, Mark DB et al: Amiodarone or an implantable cardioverter-defibrillator for congestive heart failure. N Engl J Med. 2005;352:225-237.

[2] Schwab JO, Gasparini M, Lunati M et al: Avoid delivering therapies for nonsustained fast ventricular tachyarrhythmia in patients with implantable cardioverter/defibrillator: the ADVANCE III Trial. J Cardiovasc Electrophysiol. 2009;20:663-666.

[3] Poole JE, Johnson GW, Hellkamp AS et al: Prognostic importance of defibrillator shocks in patients with heart failure. N Engl J Med. 2008;359:1009-1017.

[4] Daubert JP, Zareba W, Cannom DS et al: Inappropriate implantable cardioverter-defibrillator shocks in MADIT II: frequency, mechanisms, predictors, and survival impact. J Am Coll Cardiol. 2008;51:1357-1365.

[5] Nanthakumar K, Dorian P, Paquette M et al: Is inappropriate implantable defibrillator shock therapy predictable? J Interv Card Electrophysiol. 2003;8:215-220.

[6] Moss AJ, Zareba W, Hall WJ et al: Prophylactic implantation of a defibrillator in patients with myocardial infarction and reduced ejection fraction. N Engl J Med. 2002;346:877-883.

[7] Daubert JP, Zareba W, Cannom DS et al: Inappropriate implantable cardioverter-defibrillator shocks in MADIT II: frequency, mechanisms, predictors, and survival impact. J Am Coll Cardiol. 2008;51:1357-1365.

[8] Bailin SJ, Niebauer M, Tomassoni G et al: Clinical investigation of a new dual-chamber implantable cardioverter defibrillator with improved rhythm discrimination capabilities. J Cardiovasc Electrophysiol. 2003;14:144-149.

[9] Bansch D, Steffgen F, Gronefeld G et al: The 1+1 trial: a prospective trial of a dual- versus a single-chamber implantable defibrillator in patients with slow ventricular tachycardias. Circulation. 2004;110:1022-1029.

[10] Wilkoff BL, Cook JR, Epstein AE et al: Dual-chamber pacing or ventricular backup pacing in patients with an implantable defibrillator: the Dual Chamber and VVI Implantable Defibrillator (DAVID) Trial. JAMA. 2002;288:3115-3123.

[11] Wilkoff BL, Kudenchuk PJ, Buxton AE et al: The DAVID (Dual Chamber and VVI Implantable Defibrillator) II trial. J Am Coll Cardiol. 2009;53:872-880.

[12] Friedman PA, McClelland RL, Bamlet WR et al: Dual-chamber versus single-chamber detection enhancements for implantable defibrillator rhythm diagnosis: the detect supraventricular tachycardia study. Circulation. 2006;113:2871-2879.

[13] Wathen MS, Sweeney MO, DeGroot PJ et al: Shock reduction using antitachycardia pacing for spontaneous rapid ventricular tachycardia in patients with coronary artery disease. Circulation. 2001;104:796-801.

[14] Sweeney MO, Wathen MS, Volosin K et al: Appropriate and inappropriate ventricular therapies, quality of life, and mortality among primary and secondary prevention implantable cardioverter defibrillator patients: results from the Pacing Fast VT REduces Shock ThErapies (PainFREE Rx II) trial. Circulation. 2005;111:2898-2905.

[15] Wilkoff BL, Ousdigian KT, Sterns LD et al: A comparison of empiric to physician-tailored programming of implantable cardioverter-defibrillators: results from the prospective randomized multicenter EMPIRIC trial. J Am Coll Cardiol. 2006;48:330-339.

[16] Wilkoff BL, Williamson BD, Stern RS et al: Strategic programming of detection and therapy parameters in implantable cardioverter-defibrillators reduces shocks in primary prevention patients: results from the PREPARE (Primary Prevention Parameters Evaluation) study. J Am Coll Cardiol. 2008;52:541-550.

[17] Moss AJ, Hall WJ, Cannom DS et al: Improved survival with an implanted defibrillator in patients with coronary disease at high risk for ventricular arrhythmia. Multicenter Automatic Defibrillator Implantation Trial Investigators. N Engl J Med. 1996;335:1933-1940.

[18] Moss AJ, Hall WJ, Cannom DS et al: Cardiac-resynchronization therapy for the prevention of heart-failure events. N Engl J Med. 2009;361:1329-1338.

[19] Weber M, Block M, Brunn J et al: [Inadequate therapies with implantable cardioverter-defibrillators--incidence, etiology, predictive factors and preventive strategies]. Z Kardiol. 1996;85:809-819.

[20] Rinaldi CA, Simon RD, Baszko A et al: A 17 year experience of inappropriate shock therapy in patients with implantable cardioverter-defibrillators: are we getting any better? Heart. 2004;90:330-331.

[21] Anselme F, Mletzko R, Bowes R et al: Prevention of inappropriate shocks in ICD recipients: a review of 10,000 tachycardia episodes. Pacing Clin Electrophysiol. 2007;30 Suppl 1:S128-S133.

[22] Brugada P, Brugada J, Mont L et al: A new approach to the differential diagnosis of a regular tachycardia with a wide QRS complex. Circulation. 1991;83:1649-1659.

[23] Gunderson BD, Abeyratne AI, Olson WH et al: Effect of programmed number of intervals to detect ventricular fibrillation on implantable cardioverter-defibrillator aborted and unnecessary shocks. Pacing Clin Electrophysiol. 2007;30:157-165.

[24] Klein GJ, Gillberg JM, Tang A et al: Improving SVT discrimination in single-chamber ICDs: a new electrogram morphology-based algorithm. J Cardiovasc Electrophysiol. 2006;17:1310-1319.

Chapter 10

Current Issues in ICD SVT-VT Discrimination: Pacing for SVT-VT Discrimination

Kevin A Michael, Damian P Redfearn and
Mark L Brown

Additional information is available at the end of the chapter

http://dx.doi.org/10.5772/55047

1. Introduction

The stored electrograms (EGMs) retrieved from the ICD provide a unique and useful source of information regarding the mechanism of the underlying arrhythmia.

Current ICD algorithms discriminate VT from SVT on the basis of **passive analysis** of detected **rhythms** with positive predictive values of greater than 90% [1].

Despite this, the incidence of inappropriate therapies for SVT discrimination still remains high and varies from 16% to 31% as quoted in prior studies [2]. In many ways, the ICD bears a resemblance to a diagnostic electrophysiological study. The underlying cardiac rhythm is analysed and acted on often with the delivery of anti-tachycardia pacing (ATP) if the threshold is met. This therapeutic interaction by the ICD with the underlying arrhythmia can also be interpreted as a diagnostic manoeuvre similar to the pacing techniques employed in the electrophysiology laboratory before arriving at the diagnosis (figure 1). The success or failure of ATP to terminate the underlying rhythm may both have value.

1.1. Anti-tachycardia pacing

Anti-tachycardia pacing has been demonstrated to be a safe, effective and painless therapy in randomized controlled multicentre trials [3,4]. In the PAINFREE trial two sequences of ATP were delivered before a shock in the fast ventricular tachycardia (FVT) zone. A total of 446 FVT episodes with a mean cycle length of 301 ± 24 msec were documented in 52 patients. A total of 396 of these FVT episodes were terminated by ATP alone with an adjusted efficacy of 77% (95% CI 68% to 83%) [5]. Acceleration of the VT by ATP occurred in only 10 (4%) FVT episodes but these went on to delivery of a definitive shock aborting the episode (figure 2).

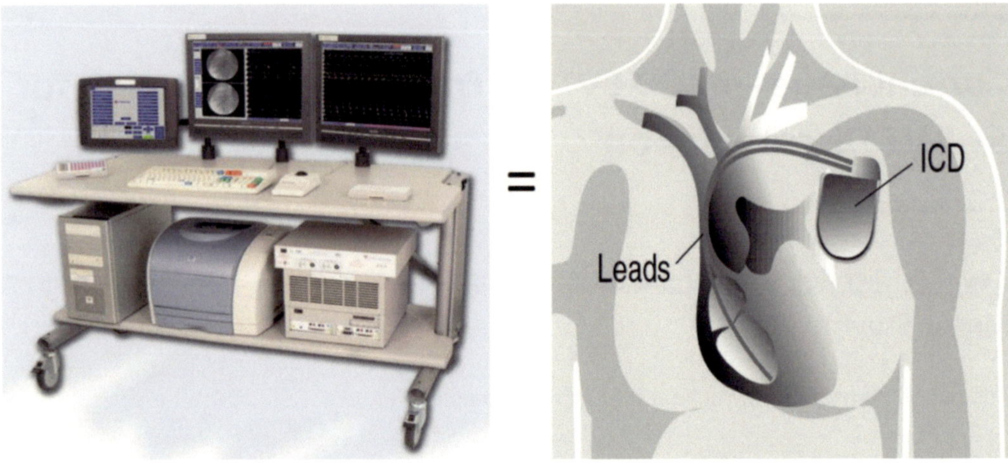

Figure 1. The ICD bears a resemblance functionally to a diagnostic electrophysiology suite

Arrhythmia related syncope that may have been from the marginal delay during delivery of ATP occurred in just 4 patients (2%) and merely involved 9 device episodes.

The PAINFREE Rx II randomized ICD patients to 2 arms: standardised empirical ATP in the FVT zone (n= 313) before shock or directly to shock in the control group (n=321) [6]. Anti-tachycardia pacing was effective in 229 of 284 episodes in the ATP arm thus yielding an adjusted efficacy of 72%. The episode duration, incidence of arrhythmic syncope and acceleration of VT was similar in both arms.

In their evaluation of ATP as first line therapy, Schoels and coworkers evaluated 760 ventricular arrhythmia episodes in 128 patients. Five hundred were appropriately detected (82 patients) [7,8].

Their analysis however showed that with conventional ICD programming and detection there were 260 episodes that were inappropriately treated. Of these 224 (57 patients) were atrial tachycardia or atrial fibrillation (AT/AF) while the remaining 36 episodes (19 patients) were due to sinus tachycardia.

This suggests that conventional device detection algorithms are prone to misdiagnosis for supraventricular arrhythmias in a significant proportion of patients. In the case of devices programmed with ATP as first line therapy it would be painless and would not result in significant morbidity. This does not hold true if there was an inappropriate shock delivered.

Since pacing is a common way of differentiating arrhythmias in an electrophysiological study, the response to this form of pacing in the ICD, by deduction may therefore hold clues as to the mechanism of the underlying detected rhythm. This then has diagnostic potential for the device specialist evaluating stored EGMs in a clinic setting and possibly has the potential for further algorithm development.

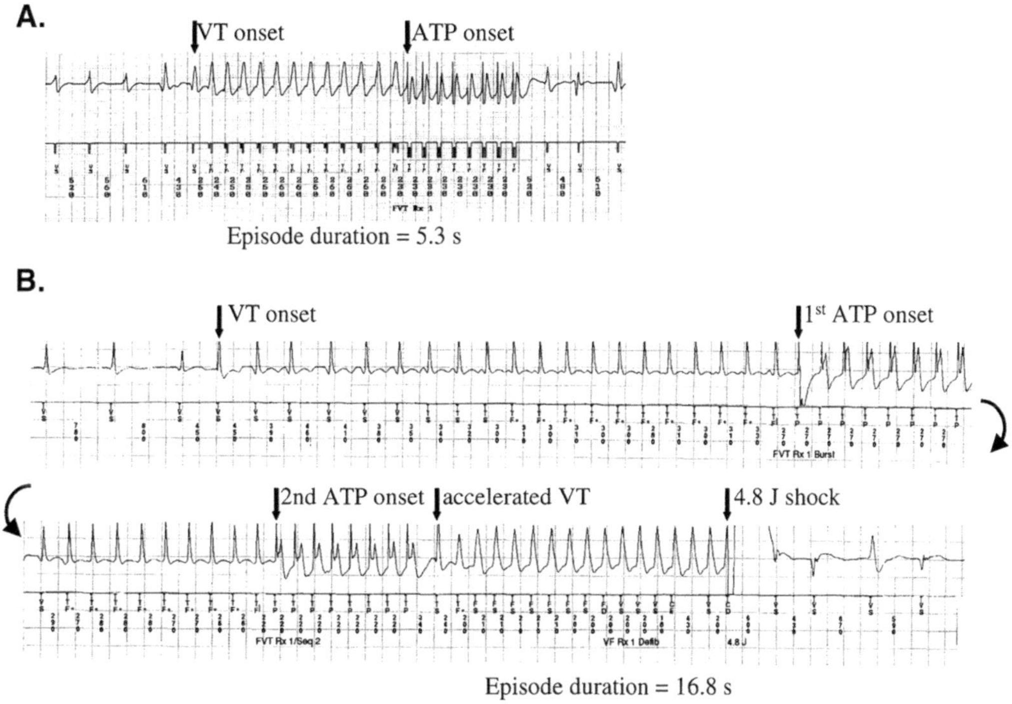

Figure 2. A. An episode of VT in the FVT zone terminated by a burst of ATP. B. The first burst of ATP in a detected VT episode fails to terminate the VT so a second burst at a shorter cycle length is delivered resulting in acceleration of the VT which then leads to a shock from the device terminating the episode.

2. Pacing to discriminate between atrial tachycardia and re-entrant SVT

Ventricular pacing and an evaluation of the atrial response after advancement of the A during retrograde conduction is a conventional manoeuvre of differentiating AT from a re-entrant SVT either AVNRT or AVRT. Knight et al. demonstrated that an A-A-V response after 1:1 VA conduction after ventricular pacing during ongoing tachycardia had a specificity and sensitivity for diagnosing AT figure 3 [9,10].

An A-V response on cessation pacing, however, suggests either AVNRT or AVRT as the underlying mechanism (figure 4). This interpretation is based on condition that the A is advanced during V pacing and that the underlying tachycardia continues unperturbed post pacing.

Using this data, it therefore seems fairly intuitive to apply these atrial responses to the interpretation of device EGMs after ATP. If there is consequent conduction to the atrium in a 1:1 fashion with advancement of the A, then the return response after pacing maybe diagnostic as discussed above [11].

This concept was applied by Ridley and co-workers to the interpretation of ICD EGMs from dual chamber ICDs (Medtronic,MN, USA) [12]. The evaluation of responses, however, was

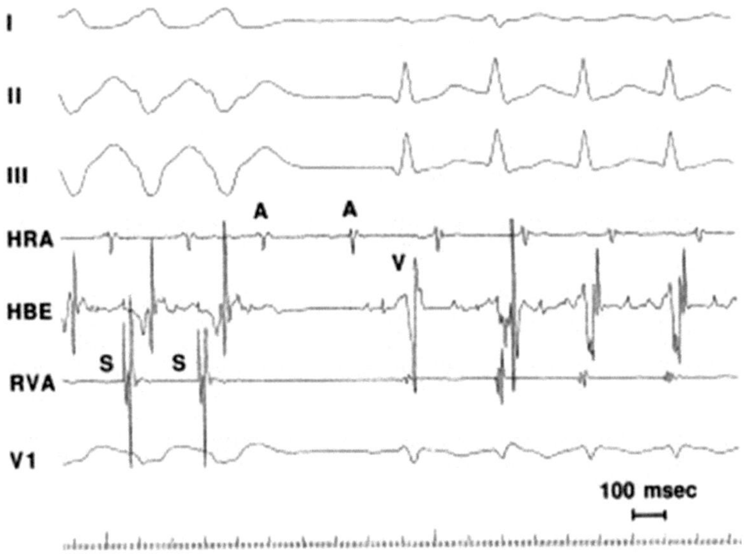

Figure 3. An A-A-V response after V pacing and 1:1 VA conduction with ongoing tachycardia suggests AT as the underlying mechanism.

based on the interval plot summary of episodes and not on the intracardiac signals. These were categorized as a type 1 response if the ventricle (V) was dissociated from the atrium (A)

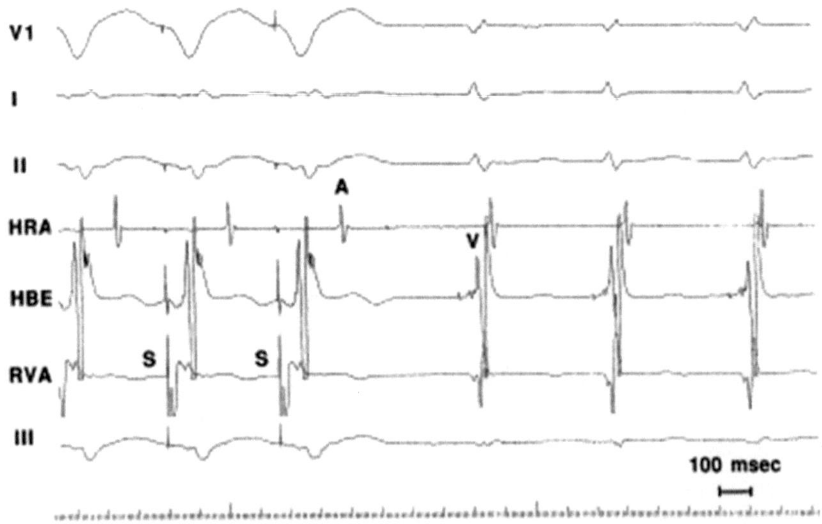

Figure 4. An A-V response on cessation of V pacing with 1:1 VA conduction suggests either AVNRT or AVRT.

http://dx.doi.org/10.5772/55047

defining the rhythm as an AT (figure 5A). A type 2 response was due to variable VA conduction and therefore leading to an inconclusive A response (figure 5B).

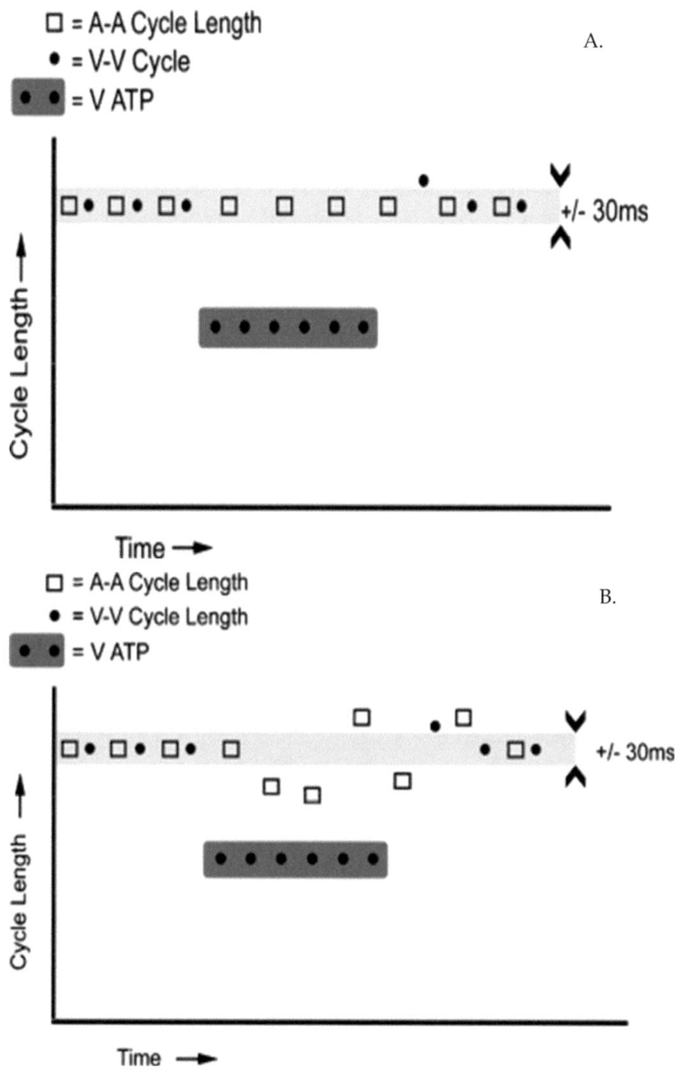

Figure 5. A. Type 1 response: the ventricular EGMs are dissociated from the atrial events during ATP. This is consistent with a diagnosis of AT. B. Type 2 response: ATP results in a variable atrial response and therefore is inconclusive.

A type 3A response occurs if the post pacing phenomenon is a V-A-A-V which is essentially an A-A-V if the last paced V, is not taken into account, as was encountered in the Knight et al. study mentioned above (figure 5C). The overall sensitivity was 71.9% (95% CI 67.1-73.6) and a specificity of 95% (95% CI 83.5-99.1). A Type 3B or V-A-V response was felt to be less conclusive for a SVT and the authors felt this did not exclude VT. This study however was based on the the interval plot as opposed to the EGMs. In our opinion, by reviewing both near and farfield EGMs in conjunction with the scatterplot, a reasonable clinical deduction can be made with regards a V-A-V response to suggest either AVNRT/AVRT. A device-based algorithm might combine pacing response with EGM morphology to discriminate the Type 3B response.

A limitation in this study was the high exclusion rate of cases since 45.1% of data could not be reliably analysed for various reasons. In 74.5% of these cases the tachycardia was terminated by the ATP as well. This, in itself, does not imply that all these episodes were VT since SVTs may also terminate with ventricular pacing. The flow diagrams in the diagnostic approach discussed later in this chapter discuss how termination of tachycardia can be evaluated to obtain a rhythm diagnosis.

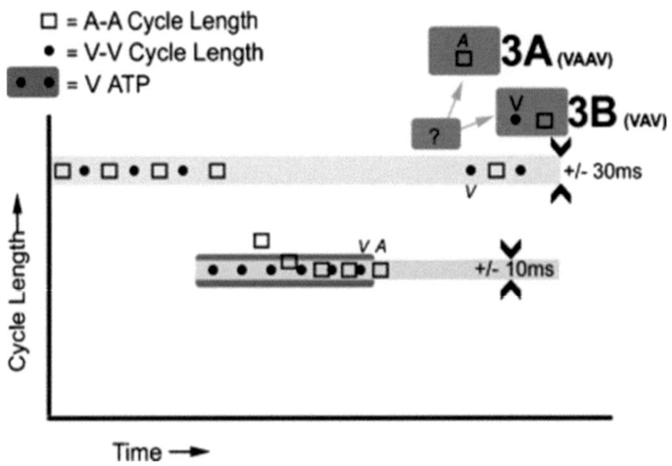

Figure 6. A type 3A response shows a VAAV pattern which is consistent with AT and a type 3B response where a VAV pattern is observed.

3. Pitfalls in interpreting the VAAV/VAV response

In order to evaluate the atrial response after V pacing, it is important to confirm that the atrium was indeed advanced during ongoing tachycardia.

Iso-arrhythmic dissociation of the ventricle at the atrial tachycardia rate may mimic 1:1 VA conduction resulting in a misdiagnosis of a VAV interval on cessation of pacing.

The next common problem is to recognise the pseudo VAAV pattern. This could occur coincidentally post ATP delivered in the ventricle with VA dissociation during an episode of AT (figure 11).

A long VA interval during an SVT as is the case in atypical AVNRT or the so called "fast-slow" variant can also yield a pseudo "VAAV" response (figure 7).

4. Limitations

The following device related limitations need to be borne in mind:

1. Over/undersensing producing an incorrect A or V response on the interval plot.

2. Timing with automatic, decaying threshold sensing may not be accurate resulting a blanking of the sensed event.

3. The 10 ms resolution in Medtronic ICDs leading to an inherent error in the estimated intervals.

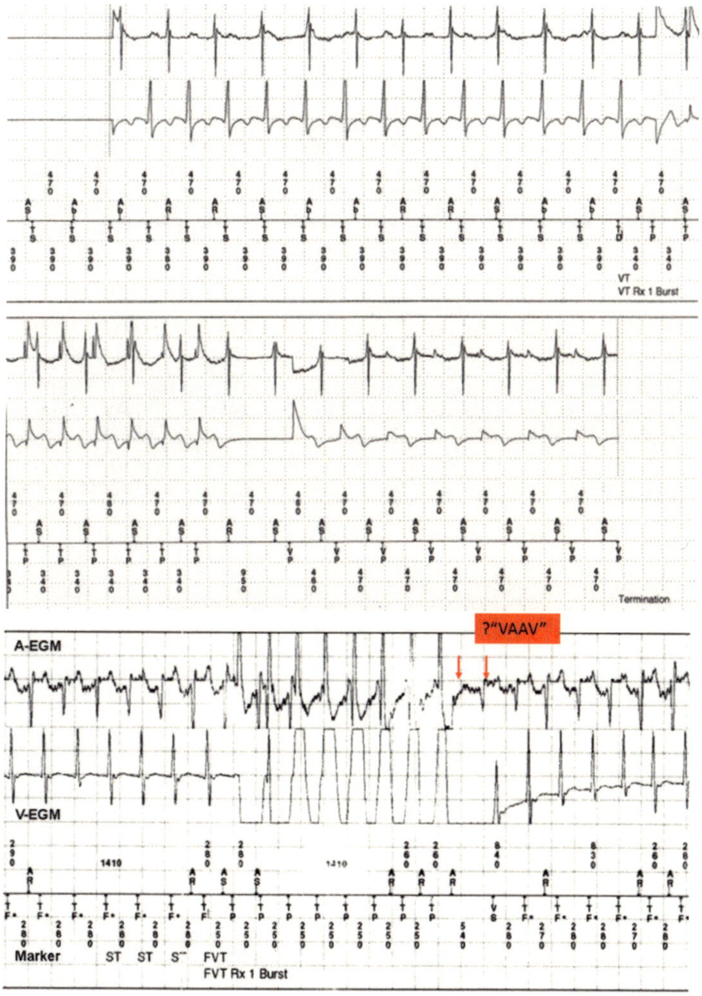

Issa, Z. F. and Mansour, I. N. J.Cardiovasc.Electrophysiol. 18(5), 548-549. 2007.

(b)

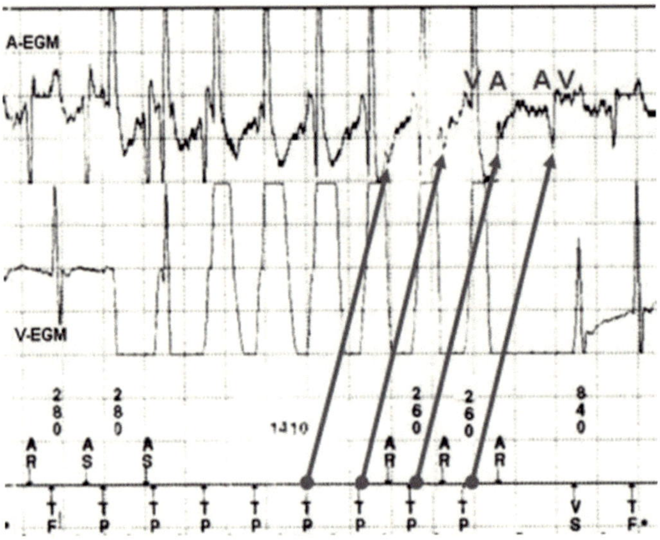

Issa, Z. F. and Mansour, I. N. J.Cardiovasc.Electrophysiol. 18(5), 548-549. 2007.

Figure 7. a). This SVT was determined to be an atypical AVNRT using a fast-slow re-entrant substrate. This was inappropriately detected and ATP was delivered by the device. On cessation of pacing a "VAAV" response is seen – or is it? (b). The same EGM is shown above. This time the arrows show each pacing spike delivered in the ventricle and the corresponding atrial signal. The last entrained atrial event (A) event is late and closer to the next ventricular sensed event(VS) because of retrograde conduction up the slow pathway. This in reality is a VAV sequence and not a VAAV response!

*1:1 Tachycardias	N:1
ST	AF
AT	Aflutter
Aflutter	AT
AVNRT	
AVRT	
VT with retrograde conduction	

*Challenge for passive ICD algorithms with variable ability to discriminate.

Table 1. Classification of Device Intracardiac EGMs

The tachycardias detected by the ICD therefore can be broadly classified as either 1:1 (A = V) tachycardias or N:1 tachycardias (ie. A > V).

The 1:1 tachycardias are difficult for both device algorithms as well as the observer to resolve as either retrograde VA conduction during VT as opposed to a SVT (table 1). However, 1:1 VA conduction only occurs in about 10% of detected VTs and therefore has a low probability [13, 14].However, the consequences of misdiagnosis of VT is much greater than the misdiagnosis of SVT. If this is misclassified as an SVT, then the result may well be a withholding of appropriate device therapies which is best avoided.

It seems rather intuitive to distinguish N:1 tachycardias as either AF, A flutter or AT if there are accompanying atrial EGMs on which to base this interpretation. Single chamber ICDs are frequently implanted if the indication is a primary prevention strategy or in the presence of persistent atrial tachycardias so that the atrial signals are lacking in these device EGMs. This then does not permit the use of algorithms that rely on A and V patterns of association in order to discriminate the rhythm. The result may well be inappropriate therapies in the form of ATP and/or shocks. It also makes it difficult for the device specialist when it comes to analysing the tracings [11].

In the example in figure 8, it is evident that the underlying arrhythmia is rapidly conducted AF. In the following clinical scenario, a single chamber ICD (figure 9), it is difficult to be certain that this is indeed an episode of VT. It may well be an organized atrial tachycardia or an episode of paroxysmal AF which is pseudo regularised and detected in tachycardia zone. Anti-tachycardia pacing is elicited as it is the first line therapy programmed in this detection zone of the device. It was deemed ineffective and therefore there was escalation to a shock. After each burst of ATP, a pause (arrows) is evident before resumption of the tachycardia. We postulated that the pause duration may help predict the chamber of origin of the tachycardia, namely VT vs AT/AF [15].

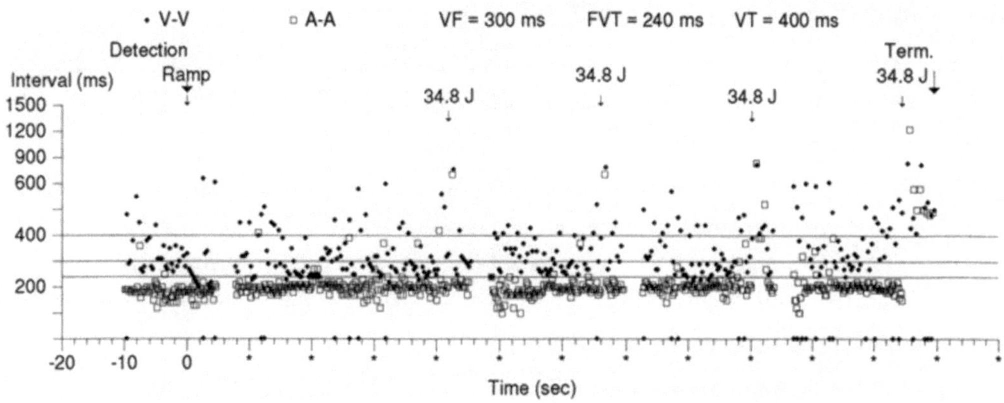

Figure 8. An interval plot showing uncontrolled atrial fibrillation detected in the VF zone of the ICD leading to ATP in the form of a ramp and then progression to sequential inappropriate shocks.

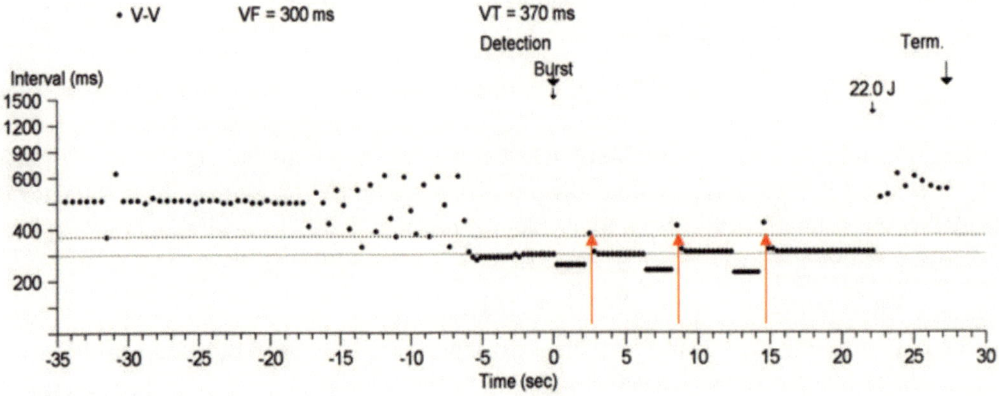

Figure 9. A treated episode in a single chamber ICD detected as VT but may also be a regular SVT with rapid onset. The absence of an atrial EGM makes it difficult to be absolutely certain.

5. The post pacing interval after ATP as discrimination tool

The mechanism of the observed pause after an episode of ATP for true VT, in fact, would represent "entrainment" provided that the VT is advanced by the ATP and then continues unchanged post ATP. This pause then can thus be referred to as the post pacing interval (PPI). The difference between the PPI and the ambient tachycardia cycle length (TCL) has been established as indication of the proximity of the pacing source to the tachycardia circuit and is a fundamental electrophysiological concept [16,17] (figure 10).

In the case of AF or AT the tachycaria source is in a relatively distant chamber, namely the atria. The pause following ATP would represent retrogarde invasion of the infra nodal conducting system and concealed penetration of the AV node.

This illustration demonstrates the concept of the PPI. After delivery of ATP and the absolute PPI and the difference between the PPI and ambient TCL (PPI-TCL) is used to predict the source of the tachycardia (figure 11).

Episodes of failed ATP for detected tachycardias in a heterogenous cohort of 250 patients receiving dual chamber and biventricular ICDs were evaluated at our centre. Fifty one events (n=18 AT/AF and n=33 VT) were eventually compared after excluding episodes in which ATP terminated or altered the TCL ≥ 50ms ie. a significant pertubation of the underlying tachycardia.

The mean PPI after failed episodes of ATP for VT and AF/AT were 512±88ms vs 693±96ms ($p<0.01$). Thus a signficant difference was observed in the pause intervals for appropriately and inappropriately delivered ATP which is understandable given the different mechanisms accounting for the PPI in each context.

http://dx.doi.org/10.5772/55047

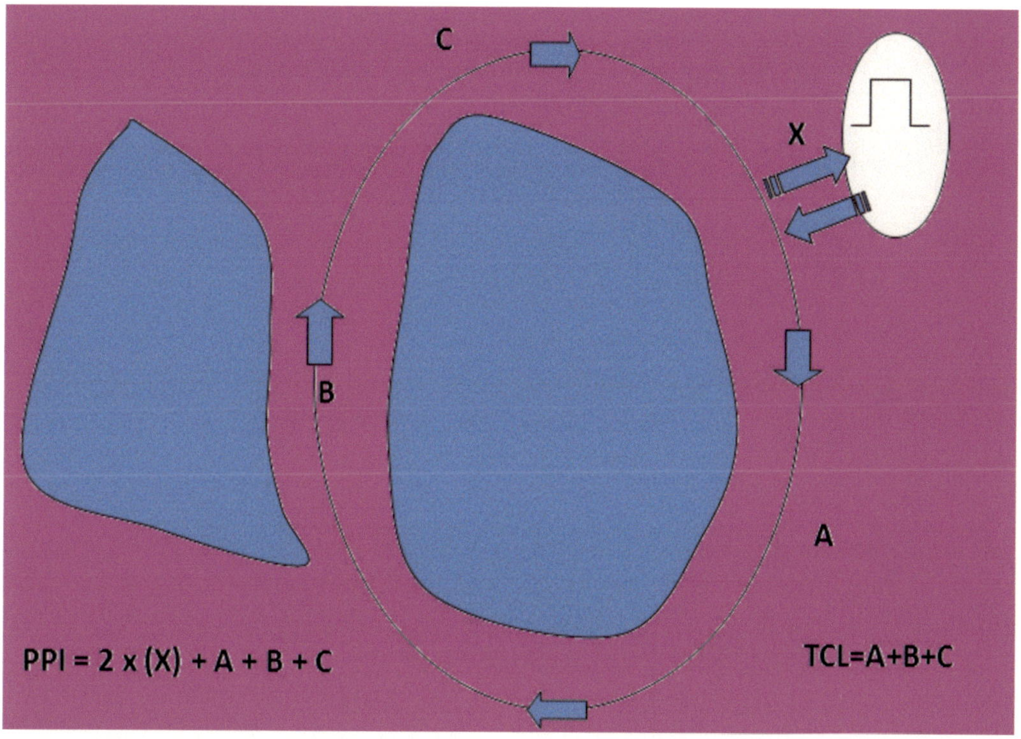

Figure 10. The pacing source is described as a distance X away from a macro-re rentrant circuit of tachycardia cycle length A +B + C. The PPI is therefore equal to the sum of 2 x X and the TCL (A+B+C).

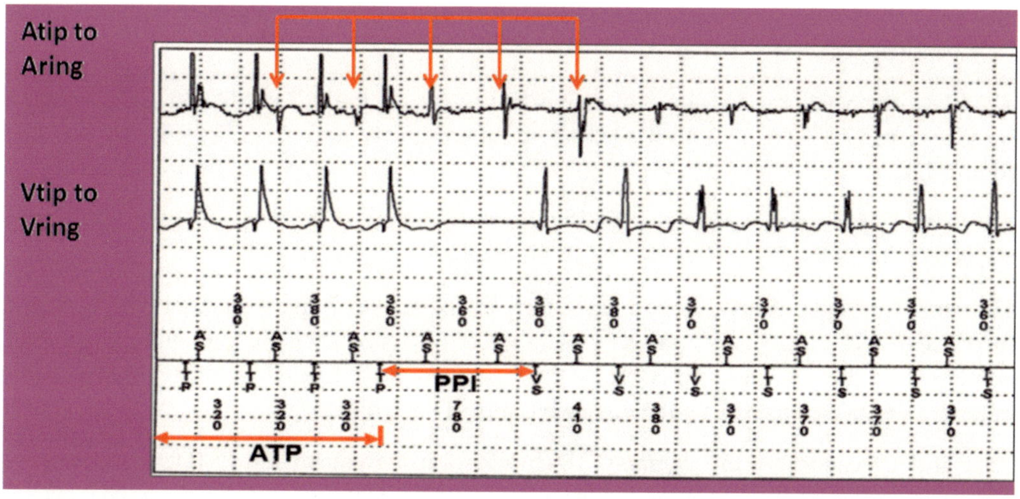

Figure 11. An episode of a 1:1 AT is inappropriately treated by the ICD. The A EGMs are dissociated from the V during ATP (arrows). There is an apparent long PPI with a pseudo VAAV response.

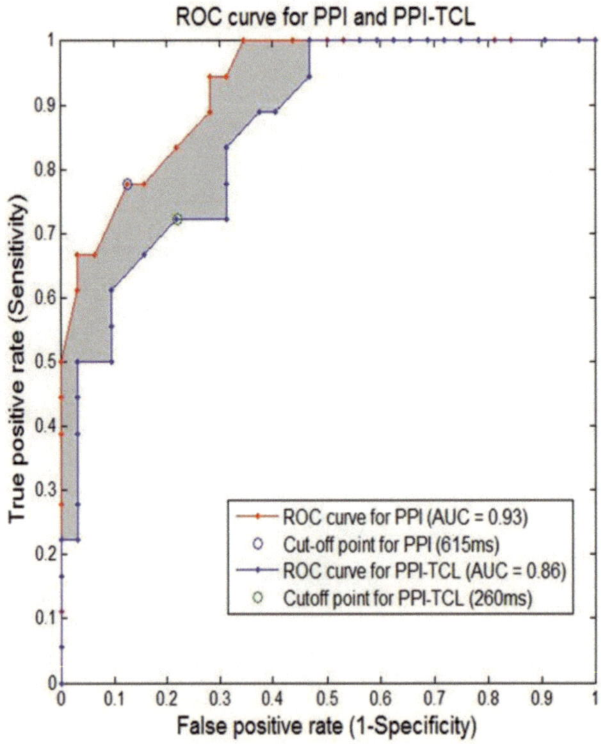

Figure 12. ROC curves for PPI and PPI-TCL and the cut-offs for each are indicated.

The same observation was made for the PPI-TCL difference for VT and AF/AT: 179±103ms vs 330±97ms ($p<0.01$), respectively.

The ROC identified cut off values of 615ms or greater for the PPI predicting AF/AT with a sensitivity of 77.8% (95% CI 58.6%-97.0%) and a specificity of 87.5% (95% CI 76.0%-99.0%) (figure 12).

A PPI-TCL ≥260ms also predicted AF/AT with a sensitivity of 72.2% (95% CI 51.5%-92.9%) and a specificty of 78.1% (95% CI 63.8% - 92.4%) (figure 12).

The use of the pause interval represents of form of active discrimination in that it relies on the response to ATP rather than a passive evaluation of EGMs which is the conventional method employed by device algorithms. This also represents a "downstream" evaluation after detection of the tachycardia by the device has already occurred.

Saba and colleagues in the Dynamic Discrimination Download Study (DD) presented a paradigm shift from the "diagnose before treating" to a "treat first and diagnose what is left" algorithm design in Medtronic dual chamber ICDs (MN, USA) [18,19]. Here, once a tachycardia was detected, ATP was applied with the delivery of 8 pulses of ATP in the atrium and ventricle.

These were delivered either simulatenously with no AV delay (SAV) or with a Covenvergent AV delay (CAV) decrementing to 0ms which was thought to be less proarrhythmic (figure 13).

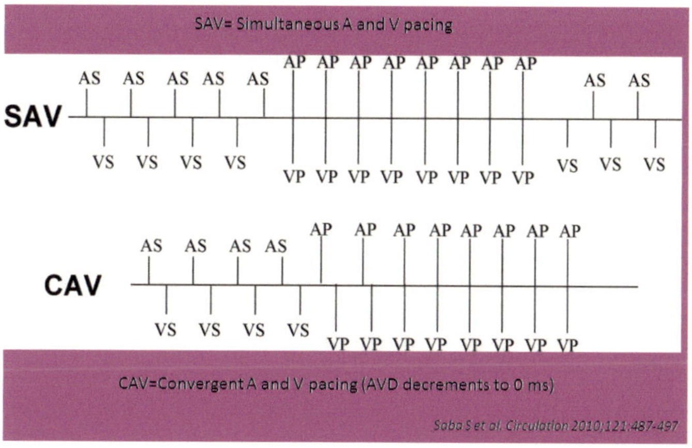

Figure 13. The two methods by which ATP was delivered in the Dynamic Discrimination Download Study (DD).

The ATP was applied initially on detection and advanced discriminators in the form of PR logic (Medtronic, MN, USA) were only applied thereafter on the remaining rhythm disorder. If the tachycardia was not terminated by ATP, the chamber in which the first sequence of tachycardia was redetected post ATP, determined whether the rhythm was classified as SVT or VT (figure 14).

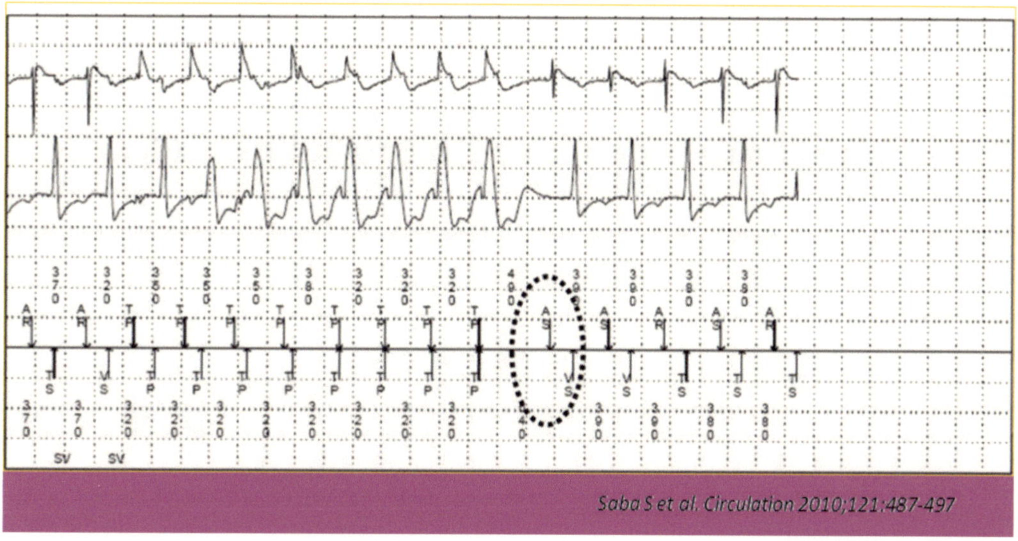

Figure 14. In this example from the DD Study, ATP is applied in the CAV (convergent AV delay) format. The tachycardia resumes post ATP with the first event being an atrial sensed (AS) EGM. This then fulfills the criteria of being an SVT.

The authors argued that if ATP terminated the tachycardia, then the time to effective therapy was shortened. If tachycardia was ongoing, then there was still no appreciable delay after the intial 8 pulses of ATP in making a definitive diagnosis. The DD algorithm terminated or correctly classified 1379/1381 SVT episodes with an overall specificity of 99.9% and 23/26 VT episodes with a sensitivity of 88.5%. There was no signficant difference in the effectiveness between the SAV and CAV ATP schemes (p>0.5). This upfront method of ATP delivery did not induce any atrial arrhythmias in the cohort studied but there was one episode of slow VT induced which spontaneously terminated.

The use of ATP as a means of pacing for SVT-VT discrimination does present some clinical challenges:

1. In the case of ventricular deliver of ATP, retrograde AV nodal conduction and advancement of the atrial EGM must be observed in order to interpret VAAV/VAV reponses.
2. ATP itself may induce premature atrial on ventricular complexes that truncate pause intervals and/or influence the assessment of the chamber of origin of tachycardia.
3. ATP must capture ventricular myocardium during the drive train.
4. ATP may accelerate or decelerate the existing tachycardia or may induce further arrhythmia.

Some possible solutions to obviate these problems would be to:

1. Deliver the ATP in multiple sequences in order to insure myocardial capture.
2. To deliver the ATP at high pacing output
3. To automatically set variable blanking periods after the delivery of ATP in order not to sense induced premature beats.

6. General considerations when approaching device based tracings

1. The chamber of onset of the tachcardia (if observed) in a dual chamber ICD has been implanted helps discriminate SVT from VT.
2. Although VT tends to be a stable rhythm, cycle length variations may occur during onset of the tachycardia or in the presence of anti-arrhythmic drugs.
3. SVTs may also present as regular tachycardias and AF may show pseudoregularisation at rapid rates.
4. If A>V events are noted this usually defines an SVT (AT, AF or A Flutter) except in the case of dual tachycadias.
5. If V>A events are noted this suggests VT although AVNRT with intermittent retrograde block should be considered but this is fairly uncommon.

http://dx.doi.org/10.5772/55047

6. 1:1 tachycardias are difficult to differentiate but VT with retrograde conduction is only observed in 10-30% of VT episodes.

These points are summarised in the following flow chart:

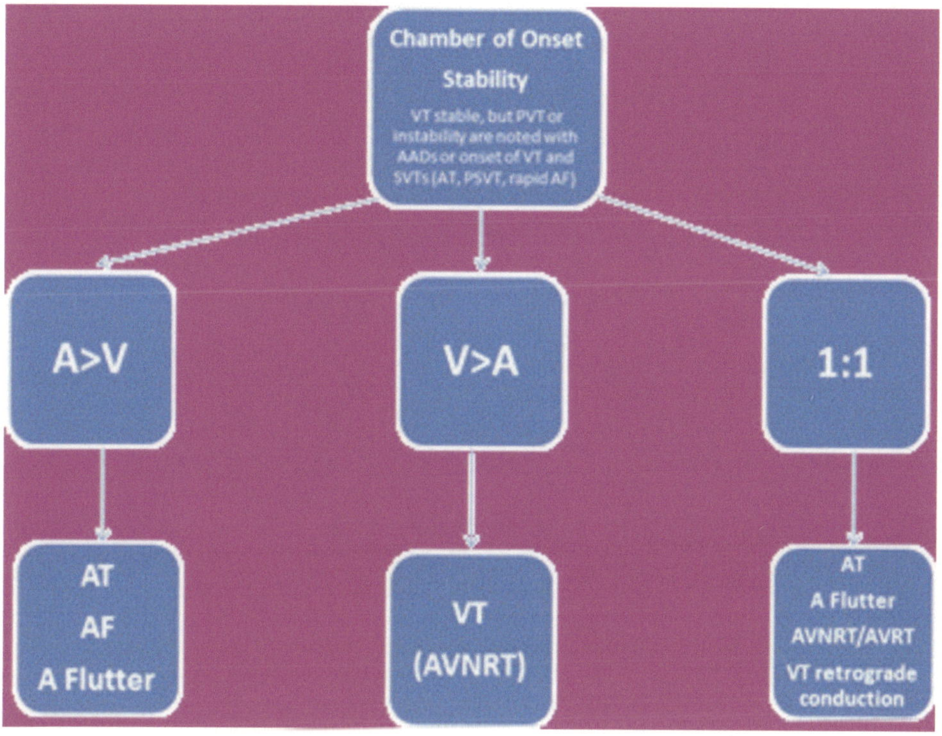

* Be aware of dual tachycardias in the A > V arm

Figure 15. A broad classification of rhythm disorders according to the A and V electrogram relationship.

In 1:1 tachycardias, the atrial EGM in dual chamber devices, during the delivery of ventricular ATP and the EGM response post ATP with ongoing tachycardia can be evaluated for the atrial response:

1. VAAV response suggests AT, unless it is a pseudo VAAV which may occur in atypical AVNRT

2. VA dissociation suggests AT

3. VAV response is compatible with AVNRT/AVRT. It does not completely rule out VT but a VVA response is suggestive of VT.

These points are summarised in the following flow chart:

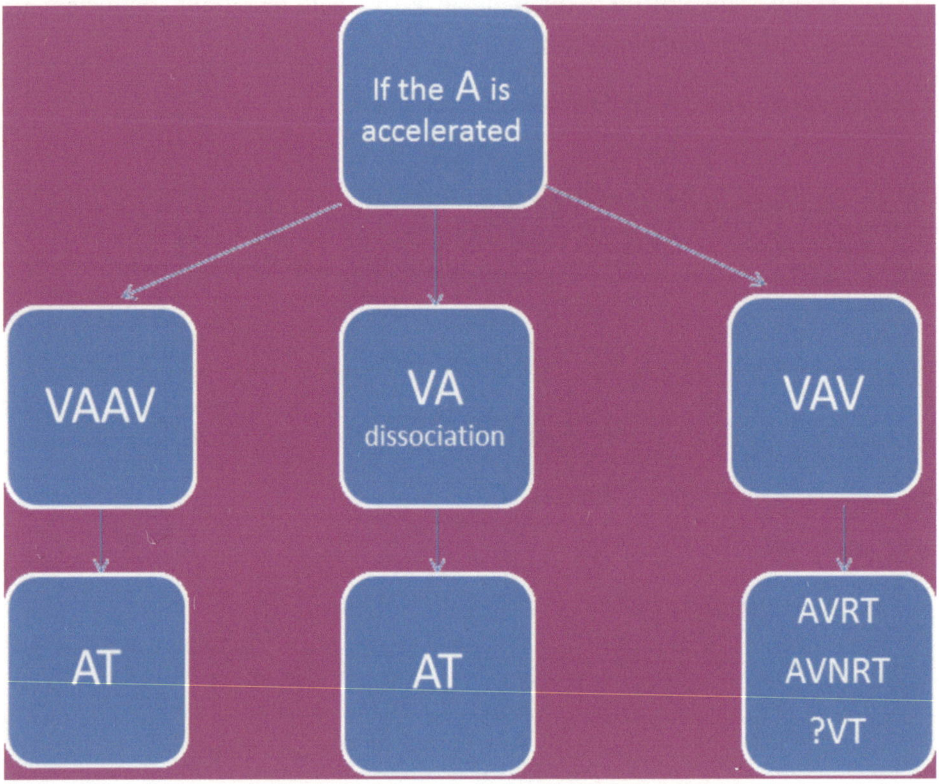

Figure 16. Arrhythmia classification based on atrial response post ATP.

Author details

Kevin A Michael[1], Damian P Redfearn[1] and Mark L Brown[2]

1 Heart Rhythm Service, Kingston General Hospital, Queen`s University, Ontario, Canada

2 Cardiac Rhythm and Disease Management Research, Medtronic, Minneapolis, USA

References

[1] Morillo CA, Baranchuk A. Deductive electrophysiology in the modern device technology era: the quest for the prevention of inappropriate ICD shocks. *J Cardiovasc Electrophysiol* 2005 June;16(6):606-7.

[2] Klein RC, Raitt MH, Wilkoff BL et al. Analysis of implantable cardioverter defibrillator therapy in the Antiarrhythmics Versus Implantable Defibrillators (AVID) Trial. *J Cardiovasc Electrophysiol* 2003 September;14(9):940-8.

[3] Sweeney MO. Antitachycardia pacing for ventricular tachycardia using implantable cardioverter defibrillators. *Pacing Clin Electrophysiol* 2004 September;27(9):1292-305.

[4] Swerdlow CD, Shehata M. Antitachycardia pacing in primary-prevention ICDs. *J Cardiovasc Electrophysiol* 2010 December;21(12):1355-7.

[5] Wathen MS, Sweeney MO, DeGroot PJ et al. Shock reduction using antitachycardia pacing for spontaneous rapid ventricular tachycardia in patients with coronary artery disease. *Circulation* 2001 August 14;104(7):796-801.

[6] Wathen MS, DeGroot PJ, Sweeney MO et al. Prospective randomized multicenter trial of empirical antitachycardia pacing versus shocks for spontaneous rapid ventricular tachycardia in patients with implantable cardioverter-defibrillators: Pacing Fast Ventricular Tachycardia Reduces Shock Therapies (PainFREE Rx II) trial results. *Circulation* 2004 October 26;110(17):2591-6.

[7] Schoels W, Swerdlow CD, Jung W et al.. Worldwide clinical experience with a new dual-chamber implantable cardioverter defibrillator system. *J Cardiovasc Electrophysiol* 2001 May;12(5):521-8.

[8] Schoels W, Steinhaus D, Johnson WB et al. Optimizing implantable cardioverter-defibrillator treatment of rapid ventricular tachycardia: antitachycardia pacing therapy during charging. *Heart Rhythm* 2007 July;4(7):879-85.

[9] Knight BP, Ebinger M, Oral H et al. Diagnostic value of tachycardia features and pacing maneuvers during paroxysmal supraventricular tachycardia. *J Am Coll Cardiol* 2000 August;36(2):574-82.

[10] Knight BP, Zivin A, Souza J et al. A technique for the rapid diagnosis of atrial tachycardia in the electrophysiology laboratory. *J Am Coll Cardiol* 1999 March;33(3):775-81.

[11] Kim MH, Bruckman D, Sticherling C et al. Diagnostic value of single versus dual chamber electrograms recorded from an implantable defibrillator. *J Interv Card Electrophysiol* 2003 August;9(1):49-53.

[12] Ridley DP, Gula LJ, Krahn AD et al. Atrial response to ventricular antitachycardia pacing discriminates mechanism of 1:1 atrioventricular tachycardia. *J Cardiovasc Electrophysiol* 2005 June;16(6):601-5.

[13] Swerdlow CD, Friedman PA. Advanced ICD troubleshooting: Part I. *Pacing Clin Electrophysiol* 2005 December;28(12):1322-46.

[14] Swerdlow CD, Friedman PA. Advanced ICD troubleshooting: Part II. *Pacing Clin Electrophysiol* 2006 January;29(1):70-96.

[15] Michael KA, Fair S, Miranda R et al. The post pacing interval following failed anti-tachycardia pacing can be used to differentiate bewteen atrial and ventricular tachycardias in ICDs. Heart Rhythm Supplement 8(5), S576. 5011.

[16] Waldo AL, Henthorn RW, Plumb VJ. Relevance of electrograms and transient entrainment for antitachycardia devices. *Pacing Clin Electrophysiol* 1984 May;7(3 Pt 2):588-600.

[17] Waldo AL. From bedside to bench: entrainment and other stories. *Heart Rhythm* 2004 May;1(1):94-106.

[18] Saba S, Barrington W, Ganz LI. New method for real-time discrimination and management of ventricular and supraventricular tachyarrhythmias applicable to patients with dual-chamber cardioverter-defibrillators. *Am J Cardiol* 2004 January 1;93(1):111-4.

[19] Saba S, Volosin K, Yee R et al. Combined atrial and ventricular antitachycardia pacing as a novel method of rhythm discrimination: the Dynamic Discrimination Download Study. *Circulation* 2010 February 2;121(4):487-97.